DR. MOERMAN'S ANTI-CANCER DIET

Holland's Revolutionary Nutritional Program for Combating Cancer

DR. MOERMAN'S ANTI-CANCER DIET

Holland's Revolutionary Nutritional Program for Combating Cancer

RUTH JOCHEMS

AVERY PUBLISHING GROUP INC.
Garden City Park, New York

The medical and health procedures in this book are based on the training, personal experiences, and research of Dr. Moerman. Because each person and situation is unique, the author and publisher urge the reader to check with a qualified health professional before using any procedure where there is any question as to its appropriateness.

The publisher does not advocate the use of any particular diet and exercise program, but believes the information presented in this book should be available to the public.

Because there is always some risk involved, the author and publisher are not responsible for any adverse effects or consequences resulting from the use of any of the suggestions, preparations, recipes, or procedures in this book. Please do not use the book if you are unwilling to assume such risk. Feel free to consult a physician or other qualified health professional. It is a sign of wisdom, not cowardice, to seek a second or third opinion.

Cover Design: Rudy Shur and Martin Hochberg
In-House Editor: Nancy M. Papritz

Library of Congress Cataloging-in-Publication Data

Jochems, Ruth, 1933–
Dr. Moerman's anti-cancer diet : Holland's revolutionary nutritional program for combatting cancer / Ruth Jochems ; foreword by Linus Pauling.
p. cm.
ISBN 0-89529-439-7 : $9.95
1. Cancer—Diet Therapy. 2. Vitamin therapy. I. Title.
II. Title: Doctor Moerman's anti-cancer diet.
RC271.D52J63 1990 90-192
616'.9940654—dc20 CIP

Printed in the United States of America

10 9 8 7 6 5 4 3 2 1

Contents

There is no shout as strong as a whisper,
as long as you whisper the truth.

Ruth Jochems

Foreword

About twenty-five years ago, my present colleague Dr. Ewan Cameron, who was then chief surgeon of Vale of Leven Hospital, Loch Lomonside, Scotland, formulated a principle that he thought could be used effectively in the control of cancer. He pointed out that people in general good health often recover from cancer, whereas those in poor general health succumb, and suggested that substances that potentiate the body's natural protective mechanisms might well provide some protection against cancer and make a significant contribution to the treatment of cancer. After having tried a number of substances without success, he began in 1971 to give 10 grams of Vitamin C per day to patients with advanced cancer, at first by intravenous infusion and then orally. It is now well known that this treatment was beneficial to almost all of the patients and of great value, extending survival time for years, to some of them.

Dr. Cornelis Moerman, in the Netherlands, had in fact formulated a similar principle many years earlier, about fifty years ago. He suggested that persons with good vitality might fight cancer more effectively than those with low vitality, and, in particular, that the vitality of a cancer patient could be greatly increased by adherence to a carefully selected diet. The evidence of his significant success over a fifty-year period is discussed in this book.

In the meantime, Dr. Moerman had trouble with the medical authorities in the Netherlands. I met Dr. Moerman about twenty years ago, and I testified in his behalf when he was under attack. Now, after half a century, he has succeeded in overcoming the opposition. In January 1987, the Ministry of Health in the Netherlands finally granted approval to his treatment.

Dr. Moerman's therapy involves eating large amounts of vegetables and fruits, and in particular drinking fruit and vegetable juices in place of water or other beverages. Bakery goods such as white bread, cake, and also foods such as macaroni and spaghetti made of white flour are forbidden. The intake of refined, white sugar is also forbidden, as well as that of meat and animal fat, other than butter. The result is that foods that are poor in vitamins and minerals are not included in the diet, which increases the supply of vitamins and minerals and other important nutrients to the patients. It is my opinion that much of the value of Dr. Moerman's therapy results from the high intake of vitamins by the patients.

In the present-day world, vitamin supplements are available at a low price, and I believe that Dr. Moerman's therapy would be improved by supplementing it with the optimum intake of Vitamin C and the other vitamins. In fact, Dr. Moerman now recommends a good intake of Vitamin C, in addition to the large amount of Vitamin C contained in the fruit juices and other foods that he recommends to the patient.

I am glad to recommend this book to cancer patients and their relatives and friends, and to others who want to improve their health with a better selection of foods.

Linus Pauling
Palo Alto, California

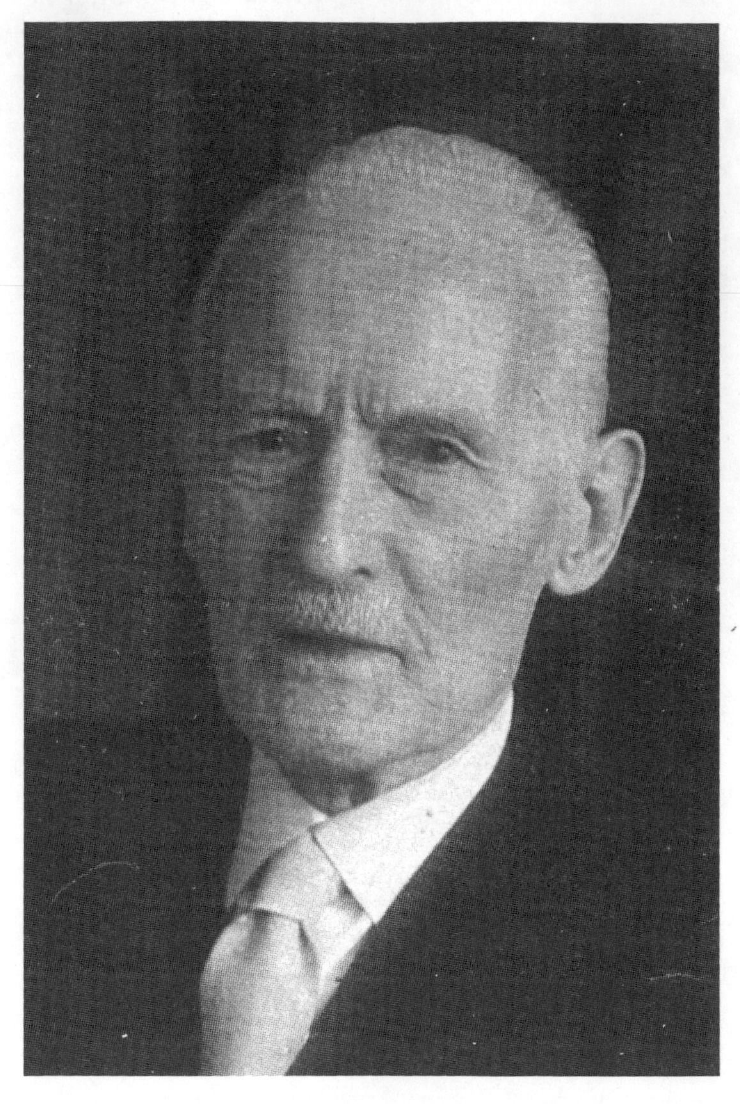

Cornelis Moerman
1893–1988

Reaching Out A Hand

Following my cancer research during the 1930s, I layed down the principles for a therapy, which, after fifty years, has lost nothing in significance. On the contrary, it has become a popular treatment, known as the Moerman Therapy, which has given relief to many cancer patients, many of whom have been cured.

The natural way of treating cancer without side effects is the most kind and human of all, thus far, known methods. It gives me satisfaction that Ruth Jochems, the author of this book, has taken my eight components regime and made it a platform for mutual worldwide cooperation between various groups practicing natural cancer treatment, to the ultimate benefit of the patient.

I hope that this admirable initiative will be crowned with the success it deserves.

Cornelis Moerman
Vlaardingen
July 15, 1988

Introduction

For more than fifty years, Holland's physicians have quietly used Dr. Cornelis Moerman's drugless diet and supplement program to treat and cure cancer. Because of its simple and inexpensive approach, it had been ridiculed by the Dutch medical, pharmaceutical, and surgical establishments since its development in 1939. This occurred despite its successful cure rate, which rivalled or surpassed so-called mainstream cancer treatments. Recently, Holland's established medical community admitted that it may have been wrong all these years.

On January 10, 1987, the Ministry of Health at The Hague—Holland's "Food and Drug Administration"—publicly recognized the Moerman Therapy as an effective cancer treatment. This government approval followed Dr. Cornelis Moerman's lifetime of striving for recognition. He died of natural causes in August 1988 at the age of 95.

On the heels of this government recognition of Dr. Moerman's nutritional attack on cancer, several of Holland's leading universities—the University of Leiden, the University of Maastricht, and the TNO at Rijswijk—reported results of rigorous clinical studies testing the relationship between diet and cancer. These university reports offered long-sought clinical proof that the Moerman Therapy was indeed sound. The findings of these reports, published recently on page one of Holland's most widely read newspaper, *De Telegraaf*, concluded that extra dietary vitamins A, C, and E would strengthen the immune system. A strong immune system would, in turn, protect the body from cancer. Dr. Moerman had been teaching precisely this—and more—for fifty years.

Although the Moerman Therapy is simple, its results are dramatic. It destroys the "ground" that cancer needs to live on by creating a "hostile" environment for cancerous cells, which is, at the same time, a beneficial environment for all existing healthy cells. By producing an anti-alkaline, well-balanced acidic, oxygen-rich body chemistry, the Moerman Therapy attacks, starves, and suffocates cancer cells while it fortifies healthy cells. As a result, tumors are encapsulated, shrink, and often disappear altogether.

The Moerman Therapy consists of two parts: a meatless, high-fiber, vitamin- and mineral-rich diet and eight supplements. Selections from the diet are substituted at mealtime. Supplements are taken at various times throughout the day. The program works without drugs. It produces no side effects. It has been used successfully both on its own and as an adjunctive therapy with immunotherapy and surgery.

The story of the Moerman Therapy began more than fifty years ago. The first patient to test Moerman's theories arrived at the doctor's doorstep in December 1939. Leendert Brinkman was suffering from a cancerous stomach tumor. In the midst of an operation to remove it, his surgeon discovered that the tumor had spread to his groin and legs. This, he said, meant that it was too late for surgery. The incision was closed. The patient was sent home to die. With nothing left to lose, Mr. Brinkman put his life in Dr. Moerman's hands.

Over the next year, he ate oranges and lemons "by the truckload," he later testified, until he was "up to his eyes in Vitamin C." Progress was slow but steady on the then-revolutionary therapeutic diet. When the year had ended, the former terminal cancer patient's body was tumor-free. He lived many more healthy years—to the age of ninety.

Motivated by his success with Mr. Brinkman, Dr. Moerman developed his ideas in greater detail. He added vitamins to acidify and oxygenate the body and a diet to fortify the immune system. He tested his theories on common park pigeons, and extrapolated results for human applications.

Soon, hundreds of case histories like Mr. Brinkman's were there for the telling. But the established medical and pharmaceutical communities were not interested in hearing them. In fact, they resisted exposure to the Moerman Therapy at every opportunity. They blocked clinical study that would prove that the program worked. They labelled Dr. Moerman a quack. The reasons for his censure were politics and greed, observers said. Dr. Moerman's enemies were other cancer researchers and powerful pharmaceutical companies. Each group stood to lose something by acknowledging Dr. Moerman's cure: the first, prestige; the second, money.

One typical adversary, a respected member of the official Dutch cancer research group, argued that the Moerman Therapy was invalid and that case histories of Dr. Moerman's patients did not offer enough proof that they were cured of cancer. Not coincidently, this spokesman had been researching his own cure, which was based on injections of radioactive iodine. His $1.5 million research grant came from the father of a 23-year-old American patient whom he had treated, but who died nevertheless one year after having been dismissed from the hospital. Clearly, this respected scientist was not about to trumpet another cure when so much rode on his own cancer research.

While researchers battled Moerman because they coveted the recognition that would come from discovering a cure, drug companies rejected or ignored the Moerman Therapy for less personal reasons. They stood to make a fortune if a "magic pill" could be found that would cure cancer. Dr. Moerman's natural, drugless approach was not something that they were interested in competing with. As a result, many of Dr. Moerman's contemporaries accused the drug industry of planting propaganda against the doctor in efforts to discredit his work.

In spite of considerable opposition, as years went by, word of the success of the Moerman Therapy spread throughout the Netherlands. Mainstream cancer specialists began to take note. Tired and disillusioned with the devastating results of chemotherapy, hormone therapy, radiotherapy, and surgery, these seasoned physicians welcomed the opportunity to offer a more gentle form of healing to cancer patients.

In the United States, Nobel prize winner Linus Pauling, at the time working on his own research with Vitamin C and cancer, became interested in the use of megadoses of Vitamin C in the Moerman Therapy. He investigated it and soon became a vocal supporter of the treatment. Dr. Pauling would eventually testify to the scientific soundness of the treatment in the midst of a maelstrom of opposition. He continues to support it, contributing the Foreword to this North American version of the Moerman Therapy.

Today, Dr. Moerman's followers continue to grow in number. In Holland alone, the 10,000 members of the Dr. Moerman association, *Moerman Vereniging,* count many cured patients among their ranks. Cure rates continue to be reported and documented. For instance, in late 1989, the Dutch Ministry of Health published a report on the results of various cancer treatments. Of a study group of 350 recovered cancer patients, 35 percent were certified cured using the Moerman Therapy alone. Of this amount, 10 patients were cured by the Moerman Therapy after having been sent home as terminal cases by orthodox medicine.

As word continues to spread of the success of this simple treatment, more cancer patients will be able to take comfort from it. It is the sincere desire of the author that the Moerman Therapy will bring help and hope to those now suffering from the pain and debilitation of solid tumor cancer. As the story on the ensuing pages tells, Dr. Moerman did indeed find a solution to the cancer riddle more than fifty years ago. The answer is simple; it is inexpensive; it is painless. It is presented here for you to use and share with those you love.

Discovery consists in seeing
what everybody else has seen
and thinking
what nobody else has thought.

Albert Szent-Györgyi

chapter one

History and Development

The story of the Moerman Therapy is one of constant refinement, dogged determination in the face of opposition, and, finally, success.

The Dutch physician Cornelis Moerman perfected his attack on cancer by continually adjusting it and comparing it to the ideas of others who strove to better understand the human body. His conclusions prove, as Albert Einstein often said, that many of the most complex problems of science would be solved simply. At the heart of the Moerman Therapy is one such solution: that changing cells' chemistry from sick to well changes a body's chemistry from sick to well because mother cells produce equal daughter cells by a process of division. Using this premise as a base, Moerman perfected a method that altered the alkaline energy supply of fermented cancer cells and produced an abundance of oxygen-rich cells at the same time. Applied to the treatment of cancer, this method—the Moerman Therapy—has achieved consistent positive results.

In the evolution of human biological science in general, and cancer therapy in particular, Cornelis Moerman must certainly be considered an important participant. Nevertheless, his work can be properly understood and valued only in the context of arising from, complementing, and supporting the discoveries of other scientists of his age.

Many of Moerman's theories are rooted in the work of Nobel prize-winning researchers who, like himself, were born at the turn of the twentieth century. Opportunities for scientific strides were rife for this generation. Born with a vista of two centuries, its members were able to view past, with its unchallenged theories and unsolved problems; present, with its wealth of better tools and technology; and future, with its heady prospect of curing the last great diseases of mankind.

Discoveries made by Moerman's contemporaries—Hungarian-American chemist Albert Szent-Györgyi, German physiologist Otto Warburg, German-British biochemist Hans Krebs, American chemist Linus Pauling, and Scottish surgeon Ewan Cameron—were essential to the formation of the Moerman Therapy.

In 1928, Szent-Györgyi isolated a substance that would become known as Vitamin C. Between 1923 and 1928, Warburg studied how the fermented chemistry of a cancer cell works. In 1953, Krebs discovered how normal cells generate energy in the presence of oxygen and citric acid. In 1971,

Pauling and Cameron reached the conclusion, on the basis of two separate arguments, that sustained megadoses of Vitamin C play a part in controlling cancer.

Moerman was among the first to combine these discoveries to create an immunity-building approach to cancer. This approach was completely different from that used by the established medical world of the day.

Formation of Basic Cancer Theories

Much of twentieth century conventional medicine bases its treatment of cancer on its acceptance of unproven assumptions of the nineteenth century. These assumptions, which comprise the following list, were first published in 1858 in the "Cellular Hypothesis" of Prussian pathologist Rudolph Virchow.

1. Cancer is a local disease.
2. The disease manifests itself by means of a tumor.
3. The tumor is comprised of abnormal cells.
4. Multiplication of those cells by division is autonomous and cannot be stopped.
5. The cells distinguish themselves by their infiltrating growth.

Today's conventional medicine continues to rely

on Virchow's theory. In fact, the most widely used forms of cancer treatment in the modern industrialized world—surgical excision, radiation, and chemotherapy—are grounded in this theory. These treatments have achieved some success in destroying tumors. But their cost to the patient in pain and suffering is enormous. Each has serious side effects. Each wears the patient down both physically and mentally. Each weakens the body's immune system. Those dedicated patients who do complete a course of chemotherapy or radiation treatment know that there is no guarantee that either of these treatments will be successful.

As long ago as the 1930s, Moerman was convinced that the natural defense systems of the human body must become the focus of attention in the search for a cancer cure. Unlike Virchow and his followers, Moerman said then, as others are admitting today, that concentrating cancer treatment on the tumor alone could not succeed.

From the beginning, Moerman rejected Virchow's theory. Instead, he said he was convinced that cancer was a manifestation of long-term environmental irritation of the body as a whole. He investigated many irritants that he felt deteriorated the body's own defense system. The most significant of these he identified as pollution, radiation, and improper nutrition. Each of these cancer promoters achieved the same end: They mutated the energy-producing deoxyribonucleic acid (DNA) of the cell, ultimately causing cancer. But, regardless of the specific cause of cancer, Moerman said, anti-cancer nutrition could reverse the course of the disease. Moerman identified the most significant of the anti-carcinogenic nutrients as Vitamins A, C, and E. These vitamins became the foundation upon which the Moerman Therapy was built.

Moerman said that continuous neglect from improper nutrition would lead to a condition of decreasing health. Decreasing health would then gain momentum as the body adapted to a primitive form of energy production: fermentation. Whereas sound nutrition and oxygen-produced energy would build normal cells, fermentation-produced energy (or, energy produced without oxygen, using glucose for fuel) would build cancer cells. Moerman said that tumors were simply visible signs that the body as a whole had adapted to fueling itself with fermentation-produced energy. This, he said, created an environment where cancer could flourish. Simply put, Virchow's cancer was a disease of one organ; Moerman's cancer was a malfunctioning of the immune system that manifested itself outwardly on the body's weakest organ as a tumor.

Thanks to Virchow, biologists spent a considerable part of a century researching the tissue of tumors. Moerman considered that to be the wrong path, however, and instead spent his time refining his conclusions that poor immunity lay at the heart of the cancer problem.

Moerman was convinced that if the overall condition of the human body could be regarded as healthy, the immune system would be capable of destroying degenerated cancer cells. If, however, the immune system were weakened as a result of prolonged wrong nutrition, cancerous cells could win the battle. Should the immune system collapse completely, the body would be rendered at the mercy of cancer. Based on these assumptions, Moerman formed the following six ideas about cancer.

1. Cancer is not an autonomous, local disease with power to destroy the body.
2. Faulty nutrition, which has adversely influenced the metabolism, precedes the formation of cancerous tissue.
3. The formation and growth of cancerous cells is not due to an autonomous force. It is the result of faulty metabolism, fueled by faulty nutrition.
4. Cancer cannot develop in a body that is in ideal health.
5. Virchow's "Cellular Hypothesis" tackles the problem of cancer at the wrong end—the tumor. It mentions the symptoms but not the cause.
6. By focusing attention on one of the major causes—malnutrition—a solution to the cancer enigma will be found.

Armed with these theories and convinced of their soundness, Moerman began to refine his methods of cancer treatment.

The Pigeon Experiments

Moerman began his clinical research in the early 1930s in the small town of Vlaardingen, Holland. A boy who lived in the town, aware of the young doctor's affection for animals, sought help from Moerman for his sick pigeon. Although the boy's pigeon was not cured, what Moerman learned from treating it contributed greatly to his growing knowledge of cancer.

The pigeon had a cancerous tumor from which, by means of an injection needle, Moerman extracted some cancerous cells. He then injected these into the breast muscle tissue of a healthy pigeon. The sick pigeon died after several weeks, but the healthy pigeon that had been injected with cancer cells remained alive. This proved to Moerman that cancer could not be induced in a healthy pigeon. He concluded that the healthy pigeon's immune system produced a "suppressor" that fought off the intruder.

Once he had formulated his first conclusion, the next step was to discover which substances in the feed guaranteed ideal health and thus rendered the pigeon immune from cancer. Moerman knew that this discovery would be significant because pigeons require the same kind of nutrition as humans, and twenty-four pigeons have about the same metabolism as one human. Moerman reasoned that what worked for pigeons could very well work for human beings.

He studied the pigeons' reactions carefully, aware that oxidation capacity is much more strongly developed in pigeons than in humans. This was important to Moerman, as he knew that it meant that the pigeons' reactions to his planned tests would be obvious and easy to define and record.

Moerman tested his theories using controlled experiments. First, he gave all of his pigeons the same feed to bring about a uniform state of health. Then, he began to differentiate. He mixed a yeast form of B-Complex vitamins in the drinking water of Group A while he continued to give plain water to Group B. Next, he varied the nutrients in the pigeons' food. He fed Group A with wheat while he fed Group B with bread crumbs. After a few weeks of this dual diet, Moerman noted that Group A was in top shape while Group B showed signs of fatigue. By observing, it became obvious to Moerman that the oxidation process of Group B had diminished due to decreased energy production. This was the direct cause of fatigue in Group B, Moerman concluded. When the situation was remedied with diet, the signs of disease disappeared. By watching the effects of diet on both healthy and sickly pigeons, Moerman became convinced that his principles were on target.

His next challenge would be to isolate the particular nutritional elements responsible for building the immune system. By testing various substances during a period of ten years, Moerman concluded that there are eight substances of vital importance to ideal health. These substances are:

1. Vitamin A
2. B-Complex vitamins
3. Vitamin C
4. Vitamin E
5. Citric Acid
6. Iodine
7. Iron
8. Sulfur

This discovery, detailed in Chapter Two, formed the basis of the Moerman Therapy.

The First Patient

Now that he had firmly established his success with animals, Moerman's next goal was to test his theories on a human being. His problem would be to find a cancer patient who would consent to be the first to be treated according to this experimental diet. In December 1939, just such a man arrived in Vlaardingen.

Terminal cancer patient Leendert Brinkman, already given up by mainstream medicine, had heard about Dr. Moerman's success curing cancer in pigeons. Suffering from an advanced, metastatic tumor of the stomach, Brinkman was sent home by his surgeon with no hope of recovery. The terminal cancer patient agreed to adhere to Moerman's guidelines if the doctor would consent to take him into his care.

During the year that followed, Moerman treated Brinkman with a rudimentary mixture of his Eight Vital Substances, coupled with a primitive form of the dietary portion of today's version of the Moerman Therapy. This included "truckloads of oranges and lemons," Brinkman later testified.

Slowly, the patient's condition improved. Although he said that he was "up to his eyes in Vitamin C," Brinkman had two important cancer weapons to get him through the long haul: faith in his doctor and the will to succeed. At year's end, a full examination was conducted. Incredibly, Brinkman's body was tumor-free. Perhaps more incredibly, Brinkman lived for "many healthy years," Dr. Moerman said. He died at the age of ninety.

Leendert Brinkman's success was the turning point for Moerman. Here, finally, was living proof that the new Moerman Therapy could cure cancer in human beings.

Refining the Basic Approach

Following his success with Mr. Brinkman, Moerman was determined to streamline and perfect his approach. During the period between 1940 and 1950, his research was geared to find the mix of proportion, quantity, and supplement that would produce the best result. Specifically, Moerman sought to answer the following three questions.

1. What is the optimum proportional relationship and interaction between the vitamins and the minerals?

2. Which quantities of vitamins and minerals should be prescribed?
3. Which additional nutritional substances should be administered?

To help him answer these questions, Moerman administered different amounts of vitamins and minerals to the many patients who now sought his help after having heard of his success with the Brinkman case. Moerman noted with interest the effects of these vitamins and minerals. By now, he was convinced that they played a significant role in tumor reduction. In fact, he observed that the vitamins and minerals had a reversing effect on symptoms that he had by now become convinced were associated with cancer. (These symptoms are discussed in detail later in this chapter.)

For example, Moerman noticed that if he gave his patients a small amount of Vitamin A, it would have practically no effect. However, when he increased the dose little by little, telltale callouses disappeared, the patient's skin became clear, and tumors stopped growing. He found that the most effective dose of Vitamin A was as high as 50,000 International Units (I.U.) daily, although he increased this dose to 100,000 I.U. in some severe cases. He noted that Vitamin A was more effective when mixed with Vitamin D. Today, biologists know that this is because these vitamins are *synergists*: substances that work better together than they do on their own.

Moerman tried out his new treatment on patients with varicose ulcers, a painful and potentially dangerous complication of varicose veins. They followed the Moerman Diet, which included many oranges and lemons—the best sources of ascorbic acid (Vitamin C) and citric acid. The patients also took generous doses of Vitamin A, Vitamin E, and small amounts of iodine. Within six weeks, their ulcers were completely healed. Thanks to experiments like these, Moerman would gradually begin to piece together the answers to his three questions.

During this period, Moerman began to develop the dietary portion of the therapy. In developing the diet, Moerman's goal was not simply to provide all the nutrition that the body needs to stay fit and healthy. The diet strictly forbade foods that damage the body and prevent good, nutritious foods from being properly used.

The Moerman Diet is not just for cancer patients. It can be followed by any person who wants to take responsibility for his or her own good health. Healthy people who follow the diet can expect to feel stronger, resist dietary deficiencies and related diseases, and see their weight normalize over a period of months.

Identifying Seventeen Symptoms

As he continued to watch and learn, Moerman became interested not only in disease and how to cure it, but also in good health and how to maintain it. When he examined the patients who came to him, particularly those suffering from cancer, he would pay attention to the whole person, not just the headache or the tumor that had brought them to see him.

As a result of his years of observation, Dr. Moerman reported that cancer patients had one or more of a total of seventeen common symptoms. He was convinced that each of these symptoms was linked to a deficiency in one or more of the Eight Vital Substances.

According to Moerman, while the presence of any one of these symptoms did not necessarily indicate that cancer was present in an otherwise healthy person, the risk of developing cancer would be greater for that person if several of these symptoms were evident at one time. Following is a complete list of these seventeen symptoms and the nutritional deficiencies that produce them.

1. Dry skin with considerably reduced elasticity. Associated symptoms: excessively callused foot soles, corn-edged skin pores, scale formation, and discolored facial skin. Indicates a lack of Vitamin A.
2. Aberration of the mucous membranes. Indicates a lack of Vitamin B-2 (riboflavin).
3. Chapped mouth corners. Indicates a lack of Vitamin B-2.
4. Red spots and scale-like formation on skin around nostrils. Indicates a lack of Vitamin B-2.

5. Dull, dry, brittle nails and chapped hands. Indicates a lack of Vitamin B-2.
6. Brown, furry coating on the tongue. Indicates a lack of nicotinamide, a component of the B-Complex vitamins.
7. Lifeless, thinning hair. Indicates a lack of Vitamin B-5 (pantothenic acid), a component of the B-Complex vitamins.
8. Gums that bleed easily. Indicates a lack of Vitamin C (ascorbic acid).
9. Black contusions that result from superficial impact. Indicates a lack of Vitamin C.
10. Slow healing of wounds. Indicates a lack of Vitamin C.
11. Formation of jelly-like regeneration tissue in a postoperative wound. Indicates a lack of Vitamin C.
12. Fatigue without due reason. Indicates a lack of Vitamin E.
13. Pale complexion. Indicates a lack of iron and cobalt.
14. Craving for sour food. Indicates a lack of citric acid, a clue that the body chemistry is alkaline and, therefore, a favorable environment for cancer cells.
15. Apathy, listlessness, and ailing vitality. Indicates a lack of Vitamins C and E.
16. Low energy. Indicates a shortage of Iodine and Sulfur. These substances fuel the energy factories in the cells' mitochondria, which absorb oxygen to split glucose to get energy so cells can breathe.

17. Sudden weight loss. Indicates a lack of Sulfur. Sulfur is necessary for digestion and cleansing.

A Growing Body of Proof

The first outside support for Moerman's ideas appeared when wartime records showed an interesting correlation between diet and cancer. In his 1954 essay entitled "Health and Prosperity," Dr. Wim Romijn presented data that supported the effectiveness of the dietary portion of the Moerman Therapy. Statistics compiled for this essay showed that cancer plummeted between the years 1942 and 1945—during the Nazi occupation of the Netherlands. Once the Second World War had ended, however, cancer rates were again on the rise. This phenomenon is depicted in Figure 1.1.

What factor was responsible for this dip and rise in cancer rates? According to Dr. Romijn, it was the anti-cancer effect of Adolph Hitler's compulsory diet. During the Nazi occupation of Holland, the Dutch people were forced to adhere to this strict diet. The white bread they were used to eating was replaced with corn bread and rye bread. Sugar, coffee, and tea were forbidden.

Other foods that might have supplemented the compulsory diet were simply not available during the war years. Production of margarine was halted.

Figure 1.1 Cancer Rates in Holland per 100,000 1940–1950

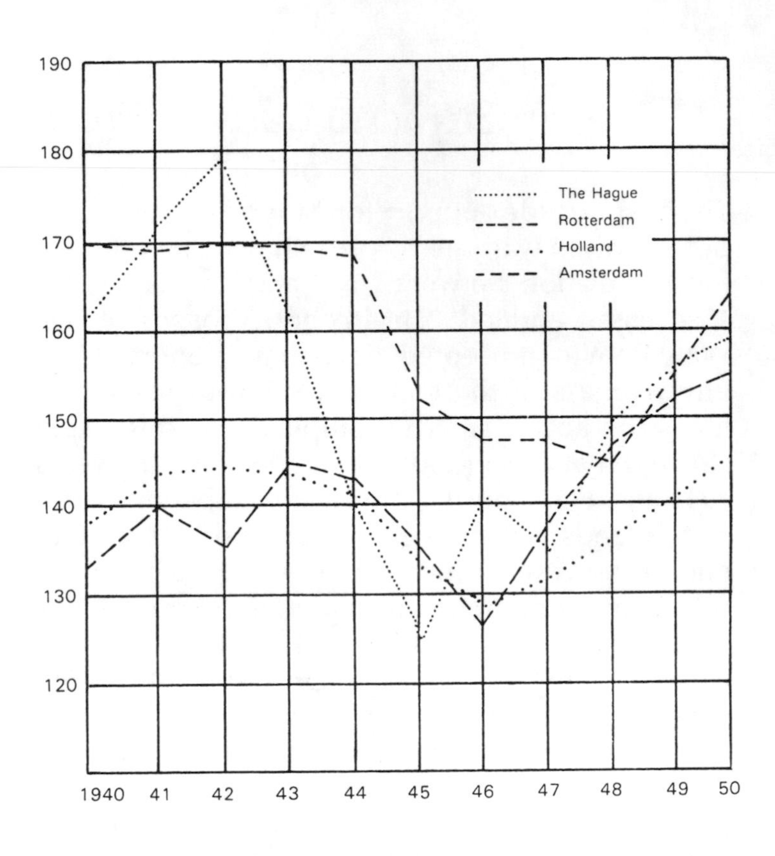

Source: Dr. Wim Romijn

Note: Numbers on left vertical represent cases per 100,000; numbers on right horizontal represent years.

Instead, there was butter—but not much of it. Alcoholic beverages were scarce luxuries. Instead, people drank fruit juices. Meat was seldom obtainable. Instead, people ate small amounts of dairy products.

Moerman's diet was remarkably similar to the wartime diet in both its ingredients and its effects. It stressed whole grains, vegetables, and fruits. It included portions of dairy products each day. It forbade such dietary villains as alcohol, coffee, meat, and tea. It had a negative effect on cancer.

Combined with the Romijn study, the testimonies of scores of Moerman's cured cancer patients offered compelling proof that diet was at the root of the cancer problem. However, Moerman's competitors and opponents all but ignored his discovery.

Moerman's Adversaries

For many decades, the politics of mainstream medicine in the Netherlands prevented Moerman's theories from being tested outright in clinical settings. This was a terrible roadblock because such tests would have lent valuable credibility to his work. All along, Moerman had proven in his own setting that cancer could be cured. Unfortunately, he knew that skeptics would need better proof. But the atmosphere of acceptance was hostile. In those sad days, knowledge that could be used for the common good was shut out to allow a relative few to profit.

Controlled by powerful men of science, universities and research hospitals closed their minds as well as their doors to Moerman's revolutionary ideas. Drug and surgical companies that were run by rich businessmen shut out Moerman's theories, as well. They chose instead to funnel huge research grants to their best customers: mainstream cancer researchers. Both groups secretly feared the doctor from Vlaardingen and other "outsiders" because they posed a threat to their orthodox way of thinking. This way of thinking benefitted both scientist and businessman.

Fierce competition between cancer researchers and their sponsor organizations to be the first to find a cure for cancer enabled drug and surgical companies to establish booming businesses as suppliers of materials, tools, and chemicals. For decades, one hand helped the other. Moerman', a country doctor not affiliated with a hospital, a university, or the business community, found no friends among his fellow cancer researchers. Limited to test and refine his theories on only those cancer patients who asked for his help, he plodded on. Ironically, fate would use Moerman's competitors to open the doors of interest to his theories.

Institute Uncovers Error in Nobel Prize Experiment

A growing number of cancer experiments conducted by Moerman's competitors disproved their own theories and instead supported Moerman's. The idea of his enemies first barring him from testing, then testing their own theories and finding that his—not their own—theories were correct must surely have filled Moerman with a renewed sense of purpose at the very least. In 1951, the Dutch Cancer Institute questioned Moerman about one such experiment, which had been conducted not long after the turn of the century.

Three rats with stomach disease were caught in a sugar refinery in Copenhagen, Denmark in 1906. They were brought to the laboratory of the noted Danish pathologist J. Fibiger. The pathologist, who according to European custom abbreviated his given name but spelled out his surname, examined the rats and pronounced that parasitic worms had burrowed through the rats' stomachs. In all three rats' stomachs, cells that had grown around the parasitic worms showed signs of abnormality. Fibiger had the sick rats examined by several independent pathologists, each of whom came to the same conclusion: Each of the rats had cancer of the stomach. This, they reasoned, was in some way caused by the worms.

Worms are common parasites in rats. They spend parts of their lives as grubs inside the bodies of cockroaches. Rats eat cockroaches. When rats eat cockroaches, they absorb the grubs inside the cockroaches, and the grubs grow to be adult worms inside the rats.

In scientific circles, Fibiger's discovery that worms had caused cancer was welcomed with great enthusiasm. It helped to back up contemporary theories that stated that all cancer was caused by some kind of long-term irritation in the body. Today, scientists call this type of long-term irritation a "trigger."

In 1926, Fibiger received a Nobel Prize for his work. But, 25 years later, his conclusions were shot down. In 1951, the Dutch Cancer Institute carried out this experiment again, but—amazingly—this time the rats did *not* get cancer. The experiment showed that the cause of cancer in these rats was not the parasitic worm acting as a trigger, but, instead, was a lack of dietary Vitamin A, which has since been proven to be an anti-carcinogen.

At a conference in the same year, the director of the Dutch Cancer Institute asked Moerman why this should be. Moerman replied that in the Dutch experiment the rats must have been fed a balanced diet, so they were able to withstand the invasion of cancer. He said that a balanced diet was important because certain substances in it had the capacity to "melt away" cancer cells and tumors. Although modern science had not yet been able to identify exactly what these substances were, Moerman predicted that they would be found to be among his Eight Vital Substances. He was proven right in both these predictions.

When Fibiger's experiments were compared with those done in Holland where the rats did not get cancer, it was discovered that the rats in Denmark had been fed bread mixed with water. By comparison, the Dutch rats' food was mixed with milk, a natural source of Vitamin A. It was the shortage of this vitamin, Moerman said, not the parasitic worm, that caused Fibiger's Danish rats to develop cancer.

Moerman did not dismiss the idea that the parasitic worm had played a role in causing cancer in the rats that were found to have it. His point was that the emphasis he placed on it was different. Fibiger and his associates and sponsors thought that they had proven that Moerman and others working along the lines of immunology were wrong by showing that the worm caused the cancer. But, ultimately, Moerman demonstrated that the *crucial* difference between the rats that got cancer and those that did not was not worms. It was their capacity to resist infection, which depended on their diet.

Today, many doctors and scientists are interested in researching which irritant factors trigger cancer. In humans, these can be environmental substances, viruses, or habits such as smoking. But what Moerman saw as the *primary* concern in cancer prevention, and what continues to be researched and investigated in the search for a cure, is the idea that the body can be reinforced to such a state of health that there are no weakened, potential cancer cells for triggers to attack.

Moerman Identifies Anti-Carcinogens

Some seventy-seven years after the Copenhagen experiments, Moerman's substances that "melt away" cancer would be given fancy names by a mainstream researcher. As Moerman predicted, one of his Eight Vital Substances would be named among them.

The first to identify substances that could attack cancer was British biochemist Sir Richard Doll, professor of medicine at Oxford University. In a series of experiments at the Dutch Cancer Institute in 1983, the Dutch biochemist L. den Engelse named these substances *anti-carcinogens*.

The Dutch study showed that anti-carcinogens work on the DNA of cancer cells by stopping the enzymatic activities of carcinogens and thereby halting their growth process. Rapid growth is the root of what makes cancer cells so dangerous. By slowing and stopping the growth of cancer cells, anti-carcinogens serve an important role in cancer treatment.

This evidence provided valuable scientific support for Moerman's work, because the research identified Vitamin A—prominent among Moerman's Eight Vital Substances—and its derivatives as important anti-carcinogens. Under a microscope, the Dutch researchers saw that Vitamin A could not only slow the growth of a cancer tumor, but that in some cases it could actually turn a malignant tumor into a benign tumor.

In today's fast-growing biotechnology industry, researchers are very interested in investigating the possibilities of using anti-carcinogens as well as genetic engineering to solve unknown mysteries of cancer. American companies and research institutes are at the forefront of these efforts. For example, at Baltimore's Johns Hopkins University, which contributes significantly to this field, young biotechnologists cannot be trained quickly enough to meet the ever-increasing outside demand for their skills.

Success With "Terminal" Patients

Based on their assumption that cancer was a tumor-specific disease, members of the orthodox medical community had traditionally "given up" on cases where cancer had spread—metastasized—beyond one organ. In their way of thinking, metastasis signified that cancer was terminal. However, mounting evidence that Moerman's theories were correct compelled mainstream researchers to investigate the stories of successful cures of so-called terminal cancer patients that were eminating from Vlaardingen.

In evaluating the Moerman Therapy, medical investigators found it extremely important to learn whether or not the Moerman Therapy was able to cure cases where cancer had spread to other organs. If this could be done, it would prove Moerman's theory that cancer was an immune-related disease, not a disease of one organ. It would then be logical to accept Moerman's premises about the relationship between diet and cancer.

According to commonly accepted conclusions about cancer, which are espoused by the Dutch Cancer Institute and many other cancer research organizations throughout the world, all mainstream cancer treatments combined are able to cure approximately 40 percent of all cancer cases. These mainstream cancer treatments include surgery, chemotherapy, radiation, radioactive iodine injections, and immunotherapy using such agents as interferon and interleukin-2. A solution is being sought for the remaining 60 percent.

While Moerman had as much success with "average" cancer patients who comprised the 40-percent category as mainstream physicians did, his most significant results were with the mainstream's so-called "terminal" cancer patients. This often desperate 60-percent category was most interested in seeking out Dr. Moerman's therapy, because mainstream methods of treatment had failed them. Of this "incurable" or "terminal" group of cancer patients, Moerman was able to cure roughly half with his diet and therapy. Documentation for these conclusions was compiled by mainstream physicians and cancer researchers who were interested in the Moerman Therapy as an alternative cancer treatment.

The SIKON Study

In 1983, several Moerman doctors formed an interdisciplinary cancer research organization, which they named SIKON. Headed by Dutch physician and Moerman doctor Jan Weise, SIKON conducted an in-depth study of the effectiveness of the Moerman Therapy. Although its study group was a relatively small 150 patients, and the study itself was done once and not repeated, SIKON's results are astonishing and cannot be ignored. The SIKON researchers presented documented proof that the Moerman Therapy achieves the same results as all other cancer therapies when used to treat common forms of solid tumor cancer. Most significant, the SIKON study showed that the Moerman Therapy is twice as effective as anything modern medicine has to offer in treating so-called terminal patients, based on a comparison of the Moerman cure rates and the 40 percent cure/60 percent "terminal" figures reported by orthodox medicine. When, in 1987, the Moerman Therapy was recognized by the Dutch Ministry of Health as a bona fide cancer treatment, SIKON's research group disbanded and its work was taken over by the Dutch Ministry of Health. Tables 1.1 and 1.2, following, show the results of the SIKON study.

Table 1.1 1983 SIKON Study Data
Solid Tumor Cancer Patients
Results by Group

Number cured with Moerman Therapy alone:	60
Number cured with Moerman Therapy after initial treatment with another therapy:	55
Total number cured with Moerman Therapy:	115
Number who could not be cured:	35
Total number in study:	150

Table 1.2 1983 SIKON Study Data
Solid Tumor Cancer Patients
Results in Percent

Percent cured with Moerman Therapy alone:	40.00
Percent cured with Moerman Therapy after initial treatment with another therapy:	36.66
Total percent cured with Moerman Therapy:	76.66
Percent who could not be cured:	23.33
Total percent in study:	99.99

However the results are interpreted, it is the author's intention to state clearly that not every case of cancer can be cured with the Moerman Therapy. However, all forms of solid tumor cancer have responded to it, and most cancer patients have found some relief in adhering to it either exclusively or as a complement to another therapy.

Latest Research Supports Moerman

Today, more is known about cancer than ever before. Much of the latest research proves that Moerman's ideas were correct. An example is new information on tumor cells. According to Drs. Ewan Cameron and Linus Pauling in *Cancer and Vitamin C*, published in 1979, tumor cells steadily release enzymes that are able to erode a way through almost every barrier placed in their path. The primary barrier is the ground substance, the intercellular "cement" of the surrounding tissue. This substance owes its high viscosity and structural cohesion to the presence of certain very large long-chain polymers, in fact macromolecules built up of endlessly repeating relatively simple molecules. The tumor cell enzyme, *hyaluronidase*, has the specific ability to break up these large polymers into shorter and shorter units. The effect of this is to liquefy the ground substance in the immediate vicinity of the tumor cells, giving them

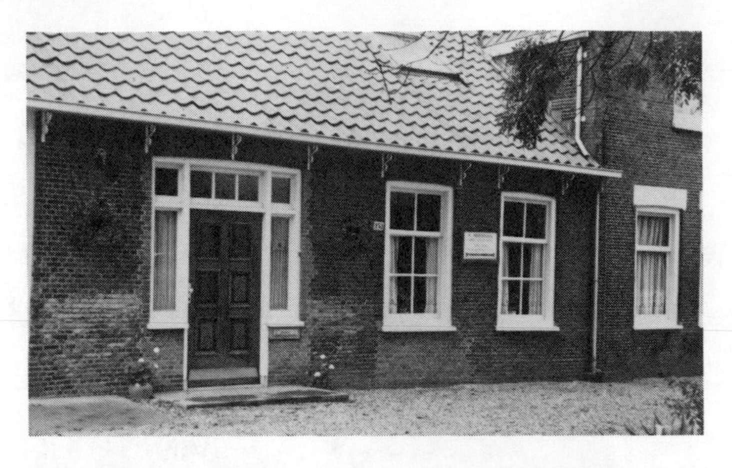

Dr. Moerman conducted his cancer research on the grounds of his family's estate. Having had no children, the doctor, who was divorced, decreed in his will that the estate be donated to his village of Vlaardingen after his death in 1988. Top photo, above, shows the doctor's home. The sign between the windows directs patients to his medical consulting room around the corner. Bottom photo, below, shows the outside structure of the family barn, where Dr. Moerman conducted his pigeon experiments. Here, Dr. Moerman collected data on nutrition and cancer that would later become the Moerman Therapy.

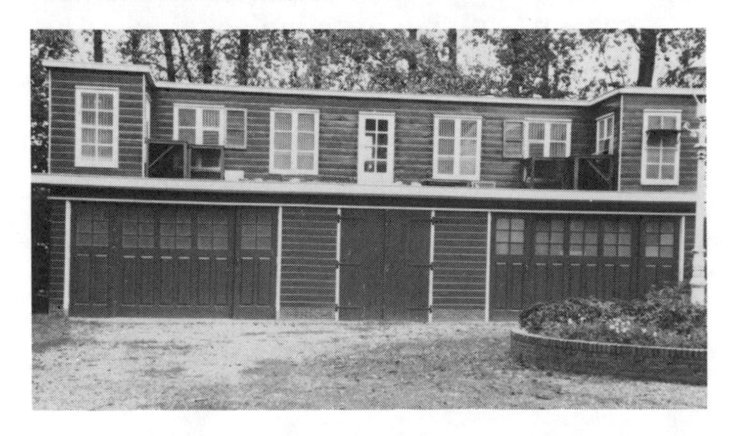

space to push forward, so the malignant cells are no longer stuck. Some drugs are known that block the action of tumor hyaluronidase, but the malignant tumors also liberate another enzyme, *collagenase,* which attacks the collagen fibrils in the ground substance, thus weakening it.

Vitamin C has the ability to strengthen this ground substance, helping it to control the disease. The effectiveness depends on improved nutrition and the use of Vitamin C supplements in proper amounts, the study says.

Readers may recall that Vitamin C has been among the Eight Vital Substances of the Moerman Therapy since the beginning, when Leendert Brinkman was instructed to eat plenty of oranges and lemons. Moerman included Vitamin C in his therapy because he said it strengthened the intercellular fibers that cancer cells so easily broke down in sickened bodies.

The Long-Awaited Seal of Approval

Though evidence mounted in support of his theories as decades passed, mainstream acceptance would continue to elude Moerman. This seal of approval was important for two reasons: It would prove that the Moerman Therapy was sound, and it would attract attention from terminal cancer patients who might not have learned of it otherwise.

Finally, on January 10, 1987, that seal of approval was granted.

Following thorough research and investigation into the Moerman Therapy, the Ministry of Health at the Hague, an organization akin to the United States Food and Drug Administration (FDA), bestowed its official seal of approval on Dr. Moerman's cancer treatment.

Although the people of the Netherlands welcomed this historic announcement in a blaze of publicity, it was not an overnight success. Cornelis Moerman's newfound fame had been hard-won, the crowning achievement of more than fifty years' work—researching, testing, and perfecting his great discovery.

Throughout Holland, the media marked the event with interviews of patients whom Dr. Moerman had cured. Representative of the group, Mr. Kappé had been told by his doctor that there was nothing he could do for him—he had cancer of the stomach and an operation was out of the question. That was eight years ago. When reporters asked Mr. Kappé's doctor to comment, all he could say was that perhaps his original diagnosis had been a bit cautious.

Case Histories

Far from a recent phenomenon, the true stories of patients cured by Dr. Moerman have been reported throughout the Netherlands for decades.

C. MOERMAN
MED. DOCTS. ARTS
SPREEKUUR
ELKE WERKDAG 1^{30}-3 uur

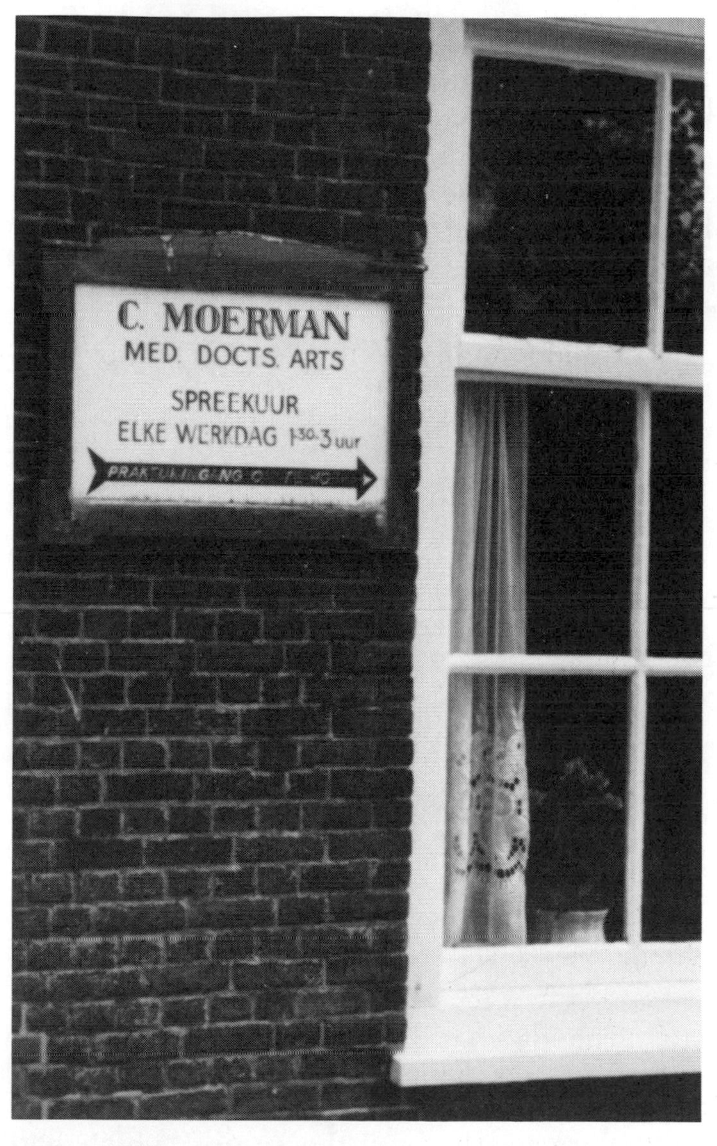

Dr. Moerman's nameplate on the front of his home served as a beacon of hope for cancer patients seeking help.

The difference is that, following its recent official government approval, the Moerman Therapy is now accepted. Examples such as those that follow have encouraged others to seek out and use the treatment.

According to the Moerman Therapy, complete healing has occurred when the following are apparent:

1. Halt of the growth of cancerous tissue,
2. Isolation of the growth of cancer to the tumor,
3. Degeneration of the ulcer.

This requires:

1. The Moerman Diet,
2. The dietary supplements,
3. An iron will to adhere exactly to the Moerman Therapy.

After following the requirements set forth, and according to the criteria for complete healing, the following representative case histories have been determined to have been cured using the Moerman Therapy.

breast cancer

Mrs. Schmidt from Rotterdam had breast cancer with metastases in the lungs. The case was considered inoperable. After a five-month treatment with the Moerman Therapy, the tumor, which had turned blueish-black, was found isolated (loose) inside the breast and the situation had improved to such an extent that the tumor could be removed with surgery. Meanwhile, the metastases in the lungs had degenerated and disappeared.

intestinal cancer

Mr. Koenig from Oud-Beyerland had a sarcoma of the connective tissue in the intestines. A tumor in his groin had grown to the size of a coconut. He had received radiation treatment five times, then was told he was incurable. After adhering to the Moerman Therapy for more than a year, both tumors began to disappear.

intestinal cancer

Mrs. Maat from Vlaardingen had been operated on to remove a malignant intestinal tumor but the tumor returned. After learning of the new tumor, her surgeon examined her and found the disease had metastasized to such an extent that a cancer specialist advised against a further operation. He referred Mrs. Maat to Dr. Moerman. Two years after, Dr. Moerman reported to the specialist that Mrs. Maat was cured.

stomach cancer

Mrs. van Oeveren from Vlaardingen visited Dr. Moerman with cancer of the stomach with numerous metastases. At the time of her initial visit, her weight had dropped to 100 pounds. She told Dr. Moerman that her surgeon said he could remove her stomach tumor but not the numerous metastases. Dr. Moerman began immediately to apply his therapy. A brief six months later, Mrs. van Oeveren had regained more than twenty pounds. At a later date, Dr. Moerman discharged her from his care. In the autumn of that year, she walked to the next village to visit a friend because, she said, "the weather was so beautiful."

Moerman Attracts Support

Over the years, many of Holland's respected physicians have accepted the Moerman Therapy as a bona fide treatment for cancer. The Dr. Moerman federation, named *Moerman Vereniging*, includes 10,000 members in the Netherlands. This group issues a list of "Moerman doctors." These physicians prescribe the Moerman Therapy for cancer patients. At present, doctors in Belgium have begun to organize and issue lists of Belgian doctors who prescribe the Moerman Therapy to hospitals in Belgium. Throughout Holland, hospital patients can choose the Moerman Therapy's diet instead of regular hospital meals. Health insurance companies in Holland now cover treatment by the Moerman Therapy in full. The program is supported by the Royal Dutch Federation of Homeopathic Doctors.

For more technical information on the Moerman Therapy, medical doctors and other interested North Americans may wish to contact the sources listed in Table 1.3, following.

Prominent Supporters Around the World

Progressive research in the fields of molecular biology, immunology, virology, and biochemistry has consistently supported the ideas that form the Moerman Therapy. As a result, prominent scien-

Table 1.3 Information Resources for the Moerman Therapy

Moerman Vereniging
(Moerman Association)
Postbox 14
NL 6674 ZG Herveld
Netherlands

President: Miss N. Ninaber
Telephone Numbers: (0)8880-1221, (0)8819-71579, (0)8370-23950

tists from around the world who work in these fields have stated that they agree with the principles of the Moerman Therapy.

Dutch geriatric specialist J. G. Defares has gone on record stating that Virchow's "Cellular Hypothesis" on cancer has become obsolete and is basically wrong.

German physician R. J. Huebner agrees with Moerman's premise that every cell of the body contains a latent virus, capable of developing cancer when the physical defense is weakened.

Nobel Laureat MacFarlane Burnet supports Moerman's thesis on immunology of the metabolism, stating that cancer results from a diminished immune system.

Both Nobel Laureat Otto Warburg and G. Domagk join Moerman in agreement that the fermentation of cells plays an active part in the development of cancer.

Two-time Nobel Laureat Linus Pauling has lauded the Moerman Therapy as "a great contribution to the solution of the cancer problem."

By building on the ideas of these men; testing, observing, and treating hundreds of cancer patients; and determining to see the battle through, Cornelis Moerman was able to achieve his lifetime goal: discovering a respected treatment for cancer.

chapter two

Principles of the Therapy

The Moerman Therapy has been carefully designed to strengthen the immune system and balance the metabolism. It is not just for cancer patients. It is also beneficial to those who wish to prepare their natural defenses before disease has had an opportunity to attack.

The regime is by no means a soft option. It is strict—but it works, and most people get used to it. Whole grain bread has more flavor and texture than white bread, and a dish of brown rice with freshly steamed vegetables and a bit of butter turns out to be very appetizing. Fruit juice instead of coffee or tea can grow on you; and you can learn to prefer the natural flavors of fresh, unprocessed foods to the added starches, chemicals, sugars, and salts of highly processed food. Chapter Three provides many creative recipes to show you what you can do with a little imagination within the restrictions of the diet.

Eating the right foods and taking the right nutritional supplements can never be the whole answer, of course. Your physical surroundings and the people around you are the keys to a positive attitude towards yourself and your health. This positive attitude is a secret weapon for beating cancer and staying well.

Cancer patients should recognize that hope and faith are vital ingredients of the cure, and the continuous success of the Moerman Therapy shows that they are always justified, no matter how dire the situation appears to be.

The chance is there for the taking, and family and friends must support the patient's decision in order to ensure the most positive outcome. Many case histories show that genuine therapeutic benefit has been gained in an atmosphere of positive thought, support, and encouragement.

The Importance of Whole Foods

Since the Eight Vital Substances that form the foundation of the Moerman Diet are all readily available from your local pharmacist, you might question whether you could take just the tablets, instead of taking the tablets as well as following the diet. The answer to your question would be that, while beneficial on their own, supplemental vitamins and minerals can never take the place of natural, whole foods. This is because fruits, whole cereals, whole grains, and vegetables always contain a balanced combination of vitamins, minerals, acids, enzymes, and fruit sugars.

Together, these elements work to digest whole foods into their most valuable and usable ingredients. Natural whole grains, for example, contain special enzymes that are necessary to digest them. These are biochemical catalysts that work to break food down into pure nutrition. There are many different enzymes. Each works to release the nutrients in the foods in which they are contained.

Modern refining methods, however, remove many of the enzymes, vitamins, and minerals in foods. This makes it harder for the body to digest and use them. For this reason, we should always eat foods that have been processed as little as possible.

Functions and Sources of the Eight Vital Substances

The Moerman Therapy focuses all regenerative energy on cancer by fueling the body with concentrated, immune-boosting nutrition in the form of whole foods and the Eight Vital Substances.

Each of the Eight Vital Substances plays an important part in keeping the body healthy. Each has an individual function and a group function. As they interact in the body, the Eight Vital Substances work together as a team to produce health. In order to understand Dr. Moerman's Therapy, it is vital to understand what these substances do and what foods they are found in. Following is an explanation of the specific functions of each of the most important nutrients contained in the Moerman Therapy.

vitamin A

This vitamin protects the skin and the mucous membranes. It is also important for the eyes—it prevents night blindness and helps weak eyesight. It is important for pregnant women to have enough Vitamin A because it is vital for the growth of the fetus. It helps to prevent acne in teenagers.

Vitamin A is found in butter, carrots, cod-liver oil, low-fat milk, spinach, and tomatoes.

vitamin B

This vitamin is, in fact, a whole group of vitamins, known as the B-Complex. The different vitamins in it are known by different names or numbers. It includes *thiamine* (B-1), *riboflavin* (B-2), *niacin* (B-3), *pantothenic acid* (B-5), *pyridoxine* (B-6), *biotin* (B-8), *folic acid* (B-9), and the *cobalamins* (B-12).

Thiamine (B-1) is necessary for the metabolism of carbohydrates, especially in the nervous system. A shortage of thiamine leads to beriberi of the nerves with muscle weakness and heart fatigue. Thiamine is found in brown rice, low-fat milk, wheat germ, and yeast.

Riboflavin (B-2) is essential to help the cells breathe properly. Brittle nails and chapped hands and lips are all signs of a deficiency. Riboflavin is found in egg yolks, green vegetables, low-fat milk, and yeast.

Niacin (B-3) helps digestion, improves circulation, reduces cholesterol levels, and maintains healthy tissue. Niacin is found in wheat germ and yeast.

Pantothenic acid (B-5) is involved in the production of hemoglobin and the breakdown of cholesterol. It is necessary for energy production. Pantothenic acid is found in broccoli, cabbage, cauliflower, egg yolks, and whole grains.

Pyridoxine (B-6) is an important member of the B-Complex vitamins. It plays a role in the metabolism of protein in the diet, and it produces a substance called *properdin*, part of the body's natural immune system. Properdin destroys bacteria and viruses in the blood. A shortage of pyroxidine affects the central nervous system and causes sleeplessness, irritability, and mood changes. Pyridoxine is found in green vegetables, whole grain cereals, and yeast.

Biotin (B-8) is essential for growth; for producing enzymes, which are necessary for digesting food; and for maintaining the body's acid balance. Skin problems, including oily skin, are caused by a lack of biotin in the diet. In healthy individuals, biotin is produced in sufficient quantity by the intestinal glands. Biotin is found in egg yolks, whole grain cereals, and yeast.

Folic acid (B-9) has been called the vitamin most lacking in American diets. It is easily destroyed when foods in which it is contained are cooked. Emotional and psychological stress destroys the body's store of folic acid. A deficiency of this B vitamin can cause chromosome damage and anemia. Folic acid is found in beets, endive, green cabbage, and whole green peas.

The cobalamins (B-12) are substances that are vital for healthy blood. Without adequate amounts of these B-Complex vitamins, anemia and tiredness can result. The cobalamins are found in egg yolks.

vitamin C

Considered a "multipurpose" vitamin, Vitamin C is perhaps the best-known of the vitamins. Vital for cell metabolism, it also helps the body to get rid of poisons. Vitamin C protects the body from the effects of harmful nitrates in cheese and meat and helps the body to absorb iron and dissolve cholesterol. It stimulates the cells that produce interferon, which fight off virus infections. Taken daily, it strengthens the immune system and reinforces the body's natural ability to heal itself.

Dr. Moerman was not the only cancer specialist to prescribe Vitamin C for his patients. Dr. Ewan Cameron, a surgeon who began his work in Scotland, was the first to experiment with it. His patients who took 10 grams of Vitamin C a day for many months achieved good results. Another firm advocate of the benefits of Vitamin C is Dr. Linus Pauling, who has written the Foreword for this book.

A lack of Vitamin C causes scurvy—weak bones and muscles, bleeding gums, and increased risk of infection.

Vitamin C is found in citrus fruits and green leafy vegetables.

vitamin E

This vitamin is important for slowing down the effects of aging. It helps to produce sex hormones in both men and women. The nervous system cannot work without it. Vitamin E helps build body tissue, muscle fiber, and blood vessels. Vitamin E is also essential for metabolism and "breathing" in the cells. It is an antioxidant, which means that it prevents fats from being destroyed by oxygen. It protects the body against cancer.

If you do not get enough Vitamin E, you may develop brown "liver spots" on your skin as you get older. Vitamin E deficiency may also lead to infertility and miscarriage. Vitamin E is found in vegetable oils, wheat germ, and whole grain cereals.

citric acid

This nutrient helps the blood to flow because it takes water from the body tissues to thin the blood. By doing this, it prevents fermentation in the cells, protects the body from blood clots, and regulates the body's acid balance. Citric acid is found in the lemon, a very important fruit in the Moerman Diet.

As well as being a rich source of Vitamin C, the lemon contains citric acid and a vitamin called citrin, also known as Vitamin P. Citrin helps the blood to flow freely through even the tiniest blood vessels. These tiny blood vessels, called capillaries, deliver blood to the skin. A shortage of citrin clogs the capillaries, and causes swollen legs, ankles, and feet.

iodine

This mineral is essential to good health even though the body requires only small quantities of it. Iodine regulates the thyroid gland, which produces the hormone *thyroxine*. Thyroxine activates the metabolism by making the cells absorb oxygen in order to burn glucose to get energy. If the mitochondria do not get enough iodine, the cells cannot get enough oxygen and they begin to ferment. As discussed in Chapter One, a fermented environment can easily breed cancer cells.

Most people get all the iodine they need from iodized salt. However, refined salt is prohibited on the Moerman Diet. Therefore, supplementation is necessary to ensure that the body has the right amount.

iron

This mineral is required for the body to produce red blood cells. Lack of iron leads to anemia. Symptoms of anemia are loss of appetite, chronic tiredness, and low immunity.

Iron is found in apricots, cherries, egg yolks, green leafy vegetables, and raspberries.

sulfur

This mineral helps the body to get rid of any poisonous materials. It is also necessary fuel for the cells' energy-producing mitochondria. Sulfur and iodine work together to ensure that the cells breathe properly.

Sulfur is found in broccoli, Brussels sprouts, cabbage, cauliflower, and egg yolks.

Directions for Taking the Eight Vital Substances

Although considerable leeway exists within the parameters of the dietary portion of the Moerman

Therapy, there is little flexibility within the parameters of the vitamin and mineral portion of the Moerman Therapy. Patients must adhere to the directions for doses, administration, and, where applicable, preparation exactly as Dr. Moerman set these down. These directions follow.

doses

In Table 2.1, doses are given in grams (g.), International Units (I.U.), milligrams (mg.), micrograms (mcg.), tablets, tablespoons, and teaspoons. Wherever doses are supplied in a range, the low-range dose should be administered to the patient with less severe symptoms; the high-range dose should be administered to the patient with more severe symptoms.

Do not administer more than the highest, high-range dose of any substance but Vitamin C. Doses higher than those supplied here, especially those shown here for Vitamin A, may be toxic. On the other hand, Vitamin C has been taken in much higher doses than those shown here without toxic side effects. Unlike the other substances in the Moerman Therapy, Vitamin C should be taken in as high a dose as is tolerated without causing stomach upset.

Table 2.1 The Moerman Therapy
Eight Vital Supplements

Element	Daily Average Dose	Daily High Range Dose
Vitamin A	50,000 I.U.	to 100,000 I.U.
B-Complex Vitamins	2 tablets	2 tablets
Vitamin C	1,250 mg.	to 5-10 g.
Vitamin E	400 I.U.	to 2,200 I.U.
Citric Acid	3 tablespoons solution	3 tablespoons solution
Iodine	3 tablespoons solution	3 tablespoons solution
Iron	3 teaspoons solution	3 teaspoons solution
Sulfur	1,000 mg.	1,000 mg.

administration

The correct timing of vitamin and mineral administration is essential to the success of the Moerman Therapy. Substances are taken according to whether they are fat-soluble or water-soluble. Vitamin A is fat-soluble and can be stored in the liver. Therefore, Vitamin A can be taken in the morning. Vitamin C, on the other hand, is water-soluble and cannot be stored in the body. Any Vitamin C that the body cannot process immediately is passed through the kidneys and is excreted from the body in the urine. Therefore, Vitamin C must be taken several times throughout the day at regular intervals to ensure the body has a constant supply.

In addition to Vitamin A, the most important fat-soluble vitamins in the Moerman Therapy are Vitamin D (supplied through the butter and egg yolks in the diet and crucial for bone tumor destruction), Vitamin E, and Vitamin K (supplied in cruciferous vegetables such as cabbage and cauliflower and helpful for blood clotting).

In addition to Vitamin C, the most important water-soluble vitamins in the Moerman Therapy are Vitamin B-1 (thiamine), Vitamin B-2 (riboflavin), Vitamin B-3 (niacin), Vitamin B-5 (pantothenic acid), Vitamin B-6 (pyridoxine), Vitamin B-8 (biotin), Vitamin B-9 (folic acid), and Vitamin B-12 (the cobalamins).

The following directions are supplied for *average* doses. Administer high range doses according to the same directions. For example, the total amount of Vitamin A should always be taken once a day; one-fifth of the total amount of Vitamin C should always be taken five times a day.

The substances should never be taken on an empty stomach. The best time to take the supplements is after breakfast with some fruit juice. Later in the day, after or between meals, the patient can take the rest of the supplements according to how many times each substance must be taken.

Table 2.2 The Moerman Therapy
Eight Vital Supplements

Element	Directions for Administration
Vitamin A	Take 50,000 I.U. once a day.
B-Complex Vitamins	Take one tablet two times a day.
Vitamin C	Take 250 mg. five times a day. (Note: Normally, cancer patients can ingest up to 10 g. of Vitamin C a day without stomach upset. The patient should take the highest dose of Vitamin C that he or she can tolerate.)
Vitamin E	Take 80 I.U. five times a day. (Note: Build up, if necessary, to 2,200 I.U. a day.) (Important: Check with your doctor if you have low blood pressure.)
Citric Acid	Take one tablespoon three times a day. Your pharmacist can prepare the following Dr. Moerman Citric Acid Solution: *Acidum citricum 10 to 15 g. with 300 g. aqua.*

Table 2.2 The Moerman Therapy
Eight Vital Supplements, continued

Element	Directions for Administration
Iodine	Take one tablespoon three times a day. Your pharmacist can prepare the following Dr. Moerman Iodine Solution: *Iodii spirit, 3%. Mix 1 to 3 drops in 300 g. water or red sour wine.* This can be prepared using equal parts of the iodii spirit and the other liquid, depending on the severity of the case.
Iron	Take one teaspoon three times a day. Your pharmacist can prepare the following Dr. Moerman Iron Solution: *Undiluted solution sacharatis ferrici aromatic triplex.*
Sulfur	Take 500 mg. two times a day: first thing in the morning, last thing at night. Your pharmacist can prepare the following Dr. Moerman Sulfur Powder: *Sulfur depuratum 0.5 g.* This powder can be mixed with butter and eaten.

Additional Considerations About Supplements

Aside from those specific dosages listed in the previous section, the following considerations should be understood before undertaking the supplement program.

children's doses

Generally, children are administered half the normal range doses of all but Vitamin C on the Moerman Therapy. The Vitamin C dose should be administered to children as listed in Table 2.3, following.

Table 2.3 The Moerman Therapy Vitamin C Dose

Age	Dose
Up to 4 years	250 mg. a day
8 years	500 mg. a day
12 years	750 mg. a day
16 years	1,000 mg. a day

vitamin B

Many doctors and patients feel that the B vitamins are simpler to buy and take in the form of the B-Complex vitamin pill. Generally, Dr. Moerman prescribed Vitamin B in this form. However, positive results have also been obtained when Moerman doctors have administered those individual B vitamins listed in Table 2.4.

Table 2.4 The Moerman Therapy Vitamin B Dose

B Vitamin	Daily Average Dose	Daily High Range Dose
B-1 (thiamine)	50 mg.	to 100 mg. a day
B-2 (riboflavin)	50 mg.	to 100 mg. a day
B-3 (niacin)	40 mg.	to 100 mg. a day
B-5 (pantothenic acid)	50 mg.	to 200 mg. a day
B-6 (pyridoxine)	20 mg.	to 100 mg. a day
B-8 (biotin)	.01 mg.	to .20 mg. a day
B-9 (folic acid)	.10 mg.	to .80 mg. a day
B-12 (cobalamin)	20 mcg.	to 100 mcg. a day

The Dietary Portion of the Moerman Therapy

In addition to understanding the functions of each of those elements that make up the Eight Vital Substances, patients should understand the following nutritional considerations when using the Moerman Therapy.

meals: timing and quantity

The essential significance of the Moerman Diet is that it is a *supplementation* to the Eight Vital Substances. Dr. Moerman was convinced that it would be useless to give a patient the Eight Vital Substances and let him or her continue to eat processed, fatty, or salty foods. This is why the Moerman Diet prohibits harmful foods. Instead, it uses mealtime as an opportunity to supply the body with as many nutrients as possible to enhance the benefits of the substances.

According to Dr. Moerman, each patient may eat according to the schedule most comfortable to him or her within the guidelines of the Moerman Diet. As explained later in this chapter, adults must eat one to two raw egg yolks each day; children must eat one raw egg yolk each day. Patients with liver or gall bladder disease should omit egg yolk from the diet until these conditions show signs of improvement, then introduce egg yolks into the diet slowly and carefully, modifying the dose according to the benefits and symptoms. Both adults and children must drink the juice of three lemons each day. Apart from these dietary laws, each patient may eat whatever mix or proportion of Moerman Diet foods he or she prefers. It is perfectly acceptable that one person will prefer to eat more vegetables and rice while another person will prefer to eat more soups and whole grain breads.

The three golden rules to remember when adhering to the Moerman Diet are:

1. Chew your food well.
2. Never eat more than you want.
3. Prepare everything carefully, so food does not lose vitamins and minerals.

Patients should eat until they are satisfied, three or more times a day. Dutch tradition dictates that one hot meal be eaten in late afternoon, but a North American patient who prefers to eat more than one hot meal a day is free to enjoy it. Table 2.5 features a sample daily menu on the Moerman Therapy.

Additional Consideration About the Moerman Diet

The dietary considerations beginning on page 56 may be significant to patients with health concerns apart from, or in addition to, cancer.

Table 2.5 The Moerman Therapy
Sample Daily Menu

Breakfast	• Juice of two oranges and one lemon • Whole grain bread with butter and cheese or • Oatmeal with fruit and low-fat milk • Buttermilk • Herb tea
Mid-morning	• Apple juice mixed with beet juice • Fruit
Lunch	• Brown rice or whole grain pasta • Steamed vegetables • Butter pat • Mixed salad with juice of one lemon and cold-pressed salad oil • Fruit
Mid-afternoon	• One or two egg yolks blended in one cup low-fat milk • Buttermilk with grape juice • Whole grain crackers

Table 2.5 The Moerman Therapy
Sample Daily Menu, continued

Supper	• Whole pea soup • Whole grain bread • Raw vegetables • Bio-Yogurt (containing dextro lactic acid only) • Fruit • Buttermilk
Late Evening	• Buttermilk with juice of one lemon
Bedtime	• Warm, low-fat milk

cholesterol

The egg yolks prescribed on the Moerman Diet are essential dietary sources of the important Vitamins A, B-1, B-2, B-6, B-12, D, and E. Egg yolks contain fair amounts of serum cholesterol, as well. Although small amounts of cholesterol are necessary to build cell walls and manufacture hormones, too much cholesterol can build up in the body causing such health problems as heart disease and stroke.

By adhering exactly to the Moerman Therapy, the body is protected from accumulating too much cholesterol. This is because the large doses of Vitamin C in the supplement portion of the

Moerman Therapy offset the doses of serum cholesterol in the diet portion of the Moerman Therapy.

laxatives

In cases where a laxative is required, one tablespoon of cold-pressed olive oil may be taken three times a day. In persistent or severe cases, the dose should be doubled.

weight gain or loss

The combination of diet and supplements in the Moerman Therapy has a beneficial effect on those who are in good health as well as those who have cancer. Normal, healthy people will lose fat with the therapy. Cancer patients may tend to gain weight. This is because the prescribed sulfur supplements cleanse the body and stimulate digestion when taken in combination with the other supplements and the foods on the Moerman Diet.

The Moerman Diet

The Moerman Diet is comprised of many foods that are easy to obtain at your local fruit and vegetable market, your local health food store, and your local grocery store. The basic ingredients of the Moerman Diet can be combined to make wholesome, healthful meals, as Chapter Three will show you.

Just as important as choosing the right foods is passing over the wrong foods. The sections on foods that comprise the Moerman Diet and on foods prohibited on the Moerman Diet that follow provide information on what to buy and what to leave on the shelf when you go shopping.

foods that comprise the Moerman Diet

The foods listed in Table 2.6 are permitted on the Moerman Diet. Feel free to use this information as your own shopping list.

The Moerman Diet: Prohibited Foods

Foods that are prohibited on the Moerman Diet contain substances that are harmful to the body under normal circumstances; potentially lethal to the body after cancer has taken hold. Salt, for example, causes the body's tissues to retain fluid. But cancerous tissues are already full of fluid. By feeding salt to cancerous tissues, a patient is not aiding the healing process. Healthy people who use the Moerman Therapy should note that any iodine that table salt would supply is provided in the supplemental portion of the program.

All foods listed in Table 2.7 are prohibited because they hinder—not help—the healing process.

Table 2.6 The Moerman Therapy: Dietary Selections

Grains

Breads, Cereals, Grains	☐ Whole grain breads ☐ Whole grain pastas ☐ Whole grain crackers ☐ Unpolished brown rice, slow-and quick-cooking varieties ☐ Barley, oat bran, wheat germ ☐ Wheat, oat, and corn flakes
Omit	■ White flour and all foods that contain white flour: breads, pastas, puddings, cakes, cookies, biscuits, gravies, sauces

Table 2.6 The Moerman Therapy: Dietary Selections

Dairy Products

Dairy Products	☐ Butter ☐ Buttermilk ☐ Cream cheese ☐ Cottage cheese ☐ Young farmer cheese ☐ Egg yolk ☐ Low-fat milk ☐ Sour cream ☐ Yogurt, plain. (Must contain dextro lactic acid, preferably with lactobacillus acidophilus Lactobacillus acidophilus restores the intestinal flora.)
Omit	■ Cheese with high fat and salt content: Bleu, Brie, Cheddar, Muenster, Swiss ■ Egg white

Table 2.6 The Moerman Therapy: Dietary Selections

Vegetables

Vegetables	□ All vegetables with the following omissions and limitations:
Omit	■ All beans and peas except whole green peas in their pods ■ All potatoes: red, sweet, white ■ Red cabbage ■ Sauerkraut ■ White cabbage
Limit	■ Brussels sprouts ■ Cauliflower ■ Green cabbage ■ Parsley
Preparation	✓Raw, organic vegetables are preferred. ✓To cook, lightly steam in water. Use no more than a pinch of sea salt in cooking water. Do not boil.

Table 2.6 The Moerman Therapy: Dietary Selections
Fruits

Fruits	☐ All fresh fruits with the following omissions and limitations:
Omit	■ Dates ■ Figs ■ Rhubarb ■ Sweet grapes
Preparation	✓ Raw, organic fruits are preferred. ✓ To cook, lightly steam in water. Use no sugar in cooking water. Do not boil. ✓ Soak all dried fruits in water for twenty-four hours; discard soaking liquid before eating.
Juices	☐ All juices of the fruits and vegetables allowed on the diet are recommended.
Highly Recommended	☐ Beet juice ☐ Carrot juice ☐ Orange juice mixed with lemon juice

Table 2.6 The Moerman Therapy: Dietary Selections

Condiments

Dressings and Seasonings	
	☐ In moderation or as otherwise indicated below.
	☐ Bay leaf
	☐ Black pepper (Limit to one pinch occasionally.)
	☐ Cream (Use occasionally.)
	☐ Garlic
	☐ Herb tea
	☐ Honey (Limit to one teaspoon daily.)
	☐ Lemon juice
	☐ Moerman Mayonnaise (Recipe in Chapter Three.)
	☐ Nutmeg
	☐ Olive oil (Use cold-pressed type only.)
	☐ Cheese, grated (Use low-fat, low-salt varieties only.)
	☐ Parsley (Use sparingly.)
	☐ Sea salt (Use only a pinch in cooking water.)
	☐ Sunflower oil (Use cold-pressed type only.)
	☐ Vegetable bouillon cubes (Use those made without chemicals or preservatives only.)

Table 2.7 The Moerman Therapy Prohibited Foods

Prohibited Foods	■ Fish ■ Meats ■ Shellfish ■ Alcoholic beverages ■ Animal fats ■ Artificial colorings ■ Beans and peas: kidney beans, lentils, marrowfat peas ■ Cheeses with high fat and salt content: Bleu, Brie, Cheddar, Muenster, Swiss ■ Chemical preservatives ■ Cigars, cigarettes, pipe tobacco ■ Cocoa ■ Coffee ■ Egg whites ■ Hydrogenated (heat-pressed) vegetable oils ■ Hydrogenated (heat-pressed) vegetable shortenings ■ Margarine ■ Mushrooms ■ Potatoes: all varieties ■ Refined, iodized table salt ■ Stocks or broths made of fish, meat, or shellfish

Table 2.7 The Moerman Therapy Prohibited Foods, continued

- Refined white sugar and all foods that contain refined white sugar: sweets, cakes, chocolates, beverages, catsup
- Teas that contain any amount of caffeine
- White flour and all foods that contain white flour: white breads, pastas, puddings, cakes, cookies, crackers, biscuits, gravies, sauces

Putting It All Into Practice

Experience and documented results prove that by combining the Moerman Therapy supplements with its diet, the cancer patient will have taken two significant steps down the road to recovery. By adding a positive outlook, the patient's chances for recovery will be enhanced further. Determination to succeed in overcoming the disease coupled with enthusiastic support from friends and family are the remaining weapons in the Moerman Therapy's attack on cancer.

The world of orthodox medicine could not ignore success stories of Dr. Moerman's patients forever. The living, breathing proof that a natural cancer cure exists has been there for all to see for more than fifty years. Although the Moerman Therapy was not something orthodox medicine was ready to accept as an effective treatment for cancer, in the end its concerned members were forced to concede that the cure rate was what counted most.

Dr. Moerman's years of devoted and painstaking research now offer hope to solid tumor patients all over the world. People once consigned to despair now have dreams for the future. These former cancer patients do not simply pay lip service to the Moerman Therapy's results: Their positive vitality attests that their faith has been justified.

The natural combination of supplement, diet, positive thought, determination, and support pioneered by Cornelis Moerman have given us a completely new approach to the problem of cancer. Thanks to his life's work, cancer is no longer the remorseless invading force, everyone's darkest fear. Now, it can be beaten; and you can win.

chapter three

Recipes

Foods that comprise the Moerman Therapy may be quite different from those that many people are used to eating. Unlike the popular fare of much of Western culture today, Dr. Moerman's menus offer no cocktails, beef steaks, or after-dinner cigars. Instead, the Moerman Therapy includes foods that, like all good fuel, burn cleanly and efficiently, adding power and vitality as they move through the system. Most patients quickly adapt to the wholesome flavors and textures, the ease of digestibility, and the sheer well-being that the diet offers. Best of all, it provides results.

The Moerman Diet consists of fresh vegetables and fruits and their juices, whole grains of all kinds, dairy products in small amounts, and natural seasonings. Though this selection might at first appear to be limited, the following basic recipes using just these ingredients illustrate that considerable variety can be achieved with a bit of imagination and a craving for good food.

Following are recipes for all sorts of wholesome things to eat: breads, spreads, sandwich fillings, soups and stews, vegetables, salads, salad dressings, sauces, main dishes, beverages, and desserts. The basic bread recipe and its variations can be made in quantity and refrigerated for several weeks. However, all of the other recipes should be made fresh and eaten immediately, as important nutrients in these recipes will be lost in refrigeration. All recipes that follow can be halved for smaller numbers of servings or doubled or tripled for larger numbers of servings, as long as these servings are eaten immediately after preparation. All fruits and vegetables must be fresh—not canned, frozen, or pre-prepared in any way. If they have not been organically grown, they should be peeled before eaten.

With these basics as your foundation, you can feel free to create your own culinary specialties using the many wholesome foods available in the dietary portion of the Moerman Therapy.

Breads

Good, healthful bread is an essential component of the Moerman Therapy. Flavor, texture, and freshness are all available from whole grain breads that are now sold at health food stores and supermarkets. But why not make your own, so that you will know exactly what it contains? The following recipe can be adapted using any whole grain flour:

wheat, rye, oat, or corn. Suggestions for variations follow the recipe.

basic recipe moerman whole grain bread

5 cups whole grain flour
1 teaspoon sea salt
1 tablespoon honey
1 1/2 cups lukewarm low-fat milk
3 teaspoons dried yeast or
6 teaspoons fresh yeast

Yield: 1 loaf

1. Mix the flour with the salt.
2. Mix the honey with the milk.
3. Dissolve the yeast in half the milk mixture and wait until it has a good, frothy head on it.
4. Add this mixture to the remaining milk mixture and add to the flour mixture.
5. Mix thoroughly to form a soft dough.
6. Knead for 5 minutes.
7. Put the dough in a warm place and leave it until it has doubled in size, about 1–2 hours.
8. Knead a second time, and place in a buttered, rectangular bread pan.

9. Leave to rise in the pan for approximately 1/2 hour.
10. Bake at 400°F for 40 minutes, until the loaf sounds hollow when knocked on the bottom. Do not over-bake.
11. Cool, slice, and serve.

variations

This basic bread recipe can be varied by adding extra ingredients to the dough before kneading. Some examples follow:

- 1 cup apricots, pitted and shredded
- 1 cup raisins
- 2 cored apples, chopped, and 1/2 cup raisins
- 4 cored apples, chopped, and 1 teaspoon cinnamon

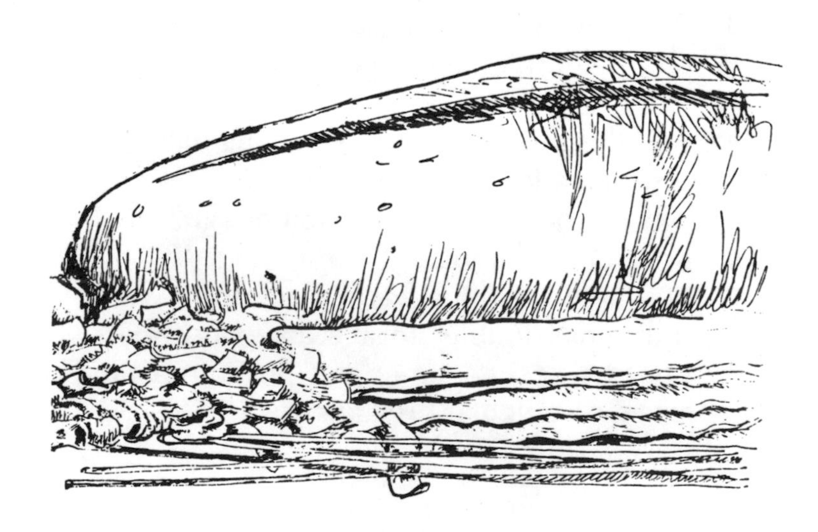

Spreads for Bread

Butter, cream cheese, cottage cheese, farmer cheese, egg yolk, sour cream, or yogurt can be blended with herbs, grated hard cheese (low-fat, low-salt varieties only), or crushed vegetable bouillon cubes to create all kinds of basic spreads. Some suggestions for variations follow the basic spread recipe, below.

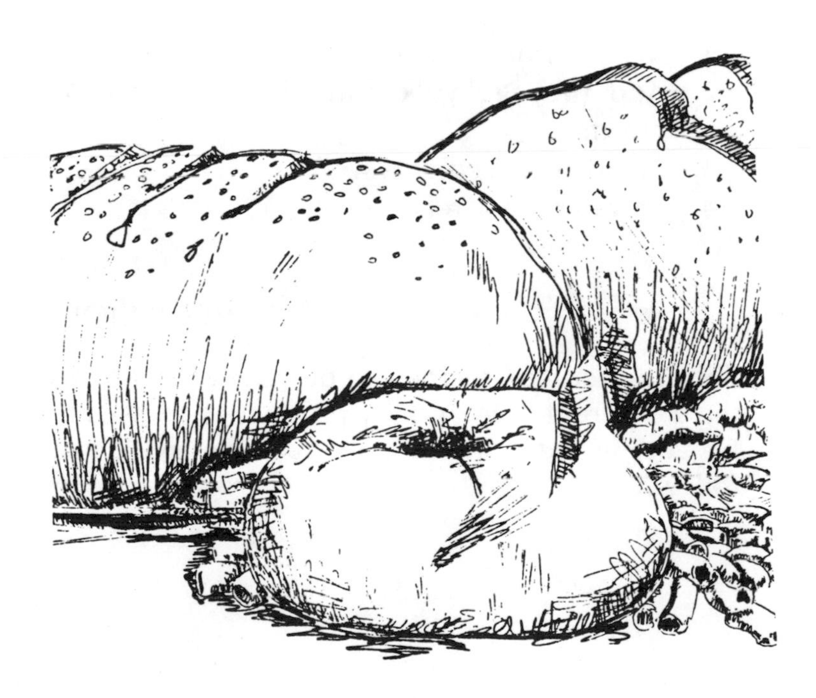

basic recipe spread for bread

1 tablespoon butter
1/2 cup grated cheese
1 egg yolk
2 tablespoons cream

Yield: 3/4 cup

1. Mix the butter with the grated cheese.
2. Add the egg yolk and the 2 tablespoons cream.
3. Blend all ingredients well.
4. Serve immediately.

variations

This basic spread recipe can be varied both by using a different type of dairy product as a base and by adding extra ingredients such as those that follow.

- 1/4 cup chopped pineapple
- 1/4 cup chopped leeks, onions, parsley, radishes, or scallions
- 1/4 cup coarsely ground hazelnuts
- 1 chopped tomato
- 1 vegetable bouillon cube, crushed
- 3 tablespoons chutney

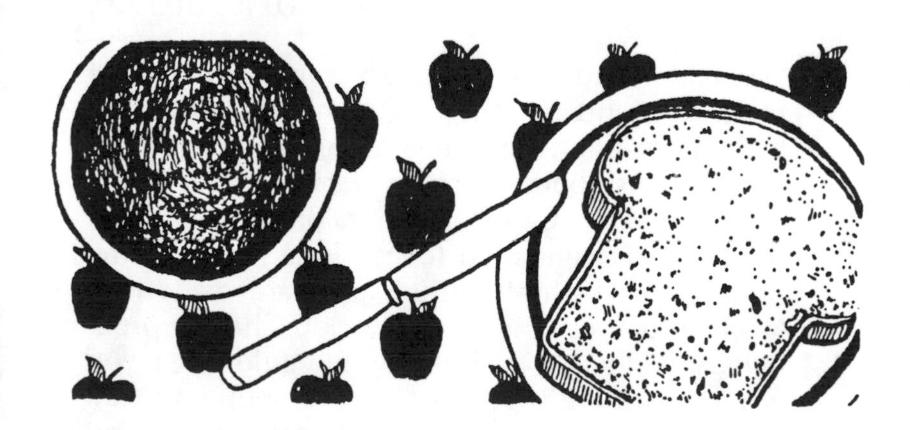

Sandwich Fillings for Bread

Almost any food on the Moerman Diet can be placed between 2 slices of whole grain bread that have been spread with a variation of the basic spread recipes to make a sandwich. Some suggestions follow.

- 1/2 cup cottage cheese mixed with the juice of 1/2 lemon, grated radishes, and chopped onions
- 1/2 cup sour cream mixed with 1/4 cup chopped scallions and 1 tablespoon fresh herbs
- 2-3 leaves watercress or lettuce sprinkled with lemon juice and topped with thin tomato slices

Soups and Stews

Vegetable soups and stews are important parts of the Moerman Diet. They are easy to prepare and make tasty, nourishing meals. For peak flavor and nutrition, use bottled spring water when a recipe calls for water. Cast-iron or stainless steel stock pots are recommended for cooking as the aluminum from which aluminum pots are made may leech into food and cause various health problems. By adhering to these simple guidelines, you will prepare the most wholesome soup you can. Suggestions for a variety of hearty soups and stews follow.

pea soup

4 cups water
4 vegetable bouillon cubes
1 1/2 cups whole, untrimmed green peas in pods (tightly packed)
3 medium onions

Yield: 4 cups

1. Combine the water and vegetable bouillon cubes in a large stock pot.
2. Wash and trim the whole peas.
3. Peel and dice the onions.
4. Combine the whole peas and the onions; bring to a boil in the vegetable broth.
5. Simmer, covered, for 15 minutes.
6. Serve immediately.

variations

This recipe may be varied by adding the following ingredients:

- Chopped basil and/or thyme, to taste
- 2–3 medium carrots, washed, peeled, and diced
- 2–3 medium leeks, washed, trimmed, and diced

tomato soup

6 large tomatoes, peeled and chopped
3 cups water
1 vegetable bouillon cube
1 medium onion, chopped
1/2 cup chopped parsley

Yield: 5 cups

1. Bring the water to a boil in a large stock pot.
2. Add the bouillon cube, the chopped onion, the chopped parsley, and the chopped tomatoes.
3. Bring to a boil; simmer, covered, for 15 minutes.
4. Serve immediately.

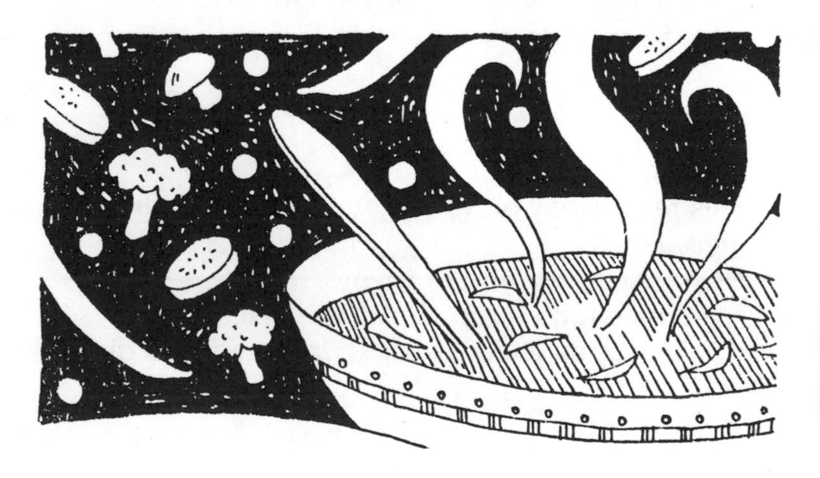

cucumber soup

1 large cucumber, diced
4 large tomatoes, peeled and chopped
1 medium onion, chopped
1 vegetable bouillon cube
1 cup water
1/2 cup grated cheese

Yield: 4 cups

1. Combine the vegetables, the vegetable bouillon cube, and the water in a covered stock pot.
2. Cook over medium heat for 15 minutes.
3. Remove from the heat.
4. Add the grated cheese and stir gently.
5. Serve immediately.

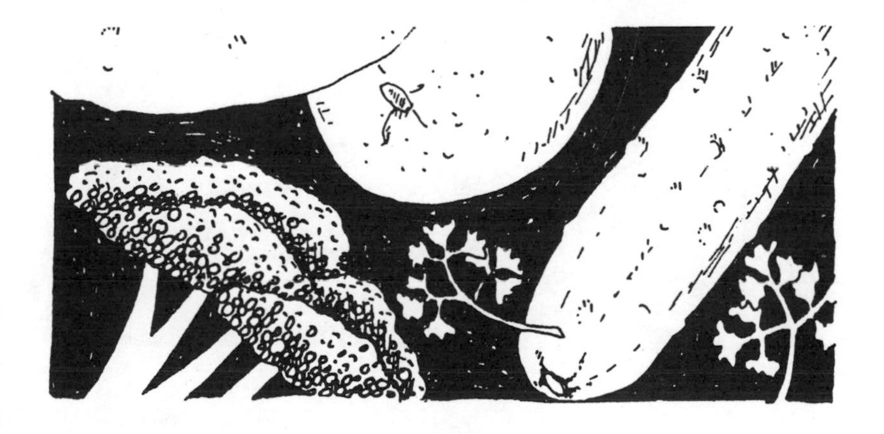

leek soup

1 medium onion, chopped
2 medium leeks, white portion only, finely sliced
3 tablespoons buckwheat
2 1/2 cups water
1 bay leaf
1 egg yolk

Yield: 3 cups

1. Combine the chopped onion, the finely sliced leeks, the buckwheat, the water, and the bay leaf in a large stock pot.
2. Simmer, covered, for 20 minutes.
3. Remove from heat, take out the bay leaf.
4. Beat the egg yolk and add to the soup, swirling the liquid as the egg cooks slightly.
5. Serve immediately.

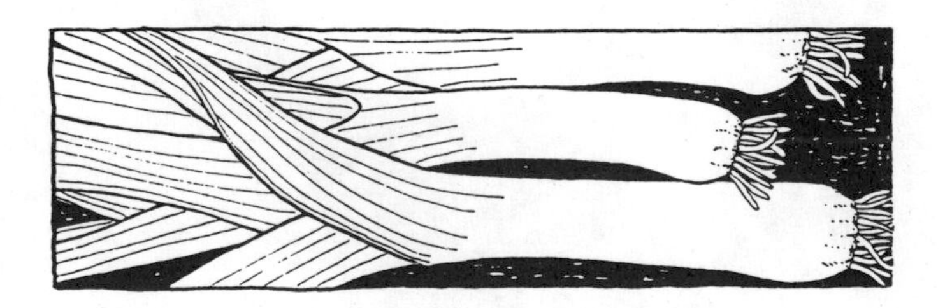

cauliflower soup

1/2 head cauliflower
1 cup water
2 cups low-fat milk
1/2 cup whole grain flour
1 vegetable bouillon cube
2 egg yolks
1/2 cup grated cheese
pinch of nutmeg

Yield: 6 cups

1. Boil the cauliflower and the water in a covered stock pot for 15 minutes.
2. Remove the cauliflower from the pot and break into chunks.
3. Make a paste of the low-fat milk, the vegetable bouillon cube, and the whole grain flour; mix this thoroughly with the water used to cook the cauliflower in the pot.
4. Bring to a boil again.
5. Reduce the heat to medium, return the cauliflower to the pot, stir.
6. Remove from the heat.
7. Beat the egg yolk and add to the soup, swirling the liquid as the egg yolk cooks slightly.

8. Serve immediately with the grated cheese on the side and a pinch of nutmeg atop each serving.

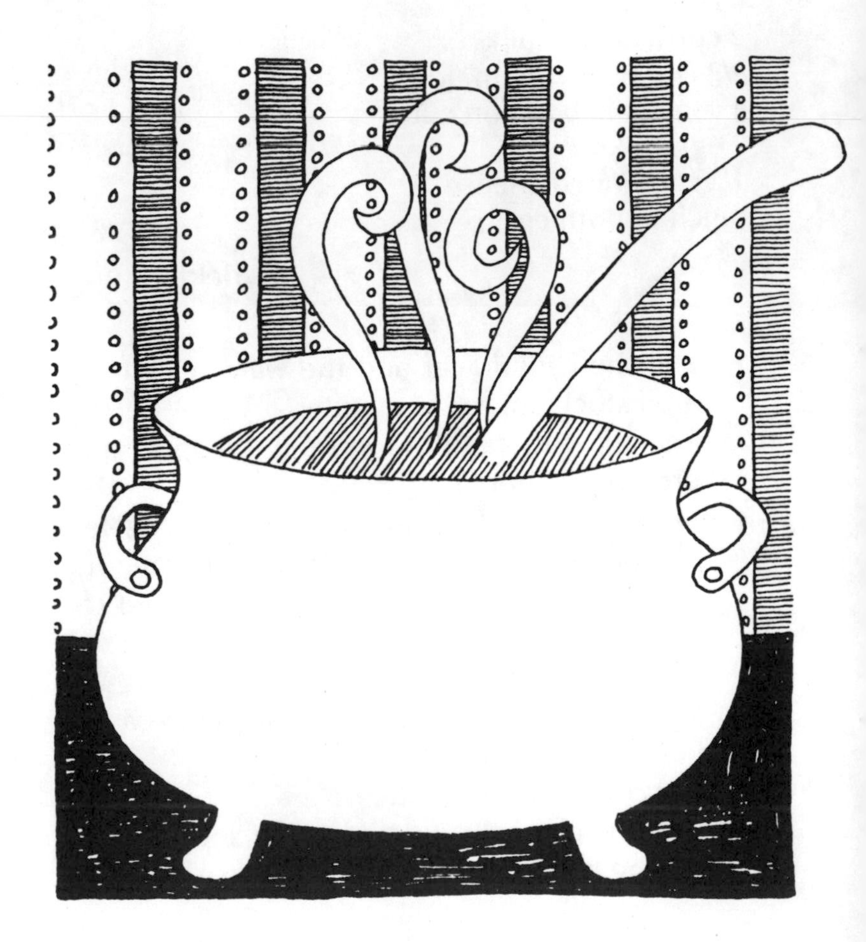

fresh vegetable broth

1 medium onion, chopped
2 medium carrots, chopped
1 medium leek, white portion only, chopped
1 large tomato, chopped
1 medium pepper, red or green, cored and chopped
1/2 cup chopped parsley
1 bay leaf
4 cups water

Yield: 6 cups

1. Combine the vegetables, the herbs, and the water in a covered stock pot.
2. Bring to a boil.
3. Turn the heat down to simmer and continue cooking, covered, for 1 hour.
4. Strain.
5. Serve the broth; discard the vegetable resins.

Vegetables

More than any other foods, fresh vegetables are the heart of the Moerman Diet. They are a valuable source of vitamins and minerals and contain the enzymes that are so vital to the healing process.

Not all vegetables are permitted on the Moerman Diet. Red and white cabbage, sauerkraut, and rhubarb must be avoided, as these can be harmful. But, the diet makes the most of the others. Full of fiber, vegetables fill us up and give us energy without making us fat. Organic vegetables are best, of course, because they have been grown without harmful fertilizers and pesticides. Home-grown organic vegetables are the best in taste, freshness, and quality.

Try, when possible, to choose vegetables that are "in season." These have not been forced to grow, but have ripened slowly, allowing nature to impart vital nutrition that is lost when vegetables are grown out of season in greenhouses. Following are some suggestions for most of North America's seasonal vegetables. Keep in mind that if your climate differs dramatically from the four seasons most of us experience your selection of seasonal vegetables will vary, as well.

spring

Asparagus, broccoli, cauliflower, chicory, cucumbers, leeks, radishes, spinach, turnips, watercress.

summer

Beets, carrots, eggplant, tomatoes, turnips, zucchini, and most of the spring vegetables.

autumn

Brussels sprouts, chicory, green cabbage, and Swiss chard.

winter

Beets, chicory, endive, parsnips, and turnips.

Cooking and Preparing Vegetables

Prepare only the number of servings of vegetables that you plan to eat immediately. Do not store cooked vegetables.

Cook trimmed and washed vegetables in as small an amount of water as possible without causing them to stick to the pan, in as little time as it takes to heat through and wilt slightly, with little or no sea salt. This cooking method will ensure that the vegetables you eat will have as much nutrition as possible. Most folks agree that vegetables taste better when they still have a bit of "bite" left in them.

Exceptions to this cooking method are made for the tough root vegetables: turnips, beets, and parsnips. These should be peeled, cubed, and boiled in an equal amount of water, in a small, covered pot, for approximately 1/2 hour, or until soft but not mushy.

Salads

Salads made from raw vegetables play an important role in the Moerman Diet. Use your imagination to provide variety. Serve salads as starters; along with the meal; or afterwards, with cheese, instead of dessert. You may add to or substitute any of the ingredients in the basic green salad recipe that follows, using any of the vegetables and fruits allowed on the Moerman Therapy.

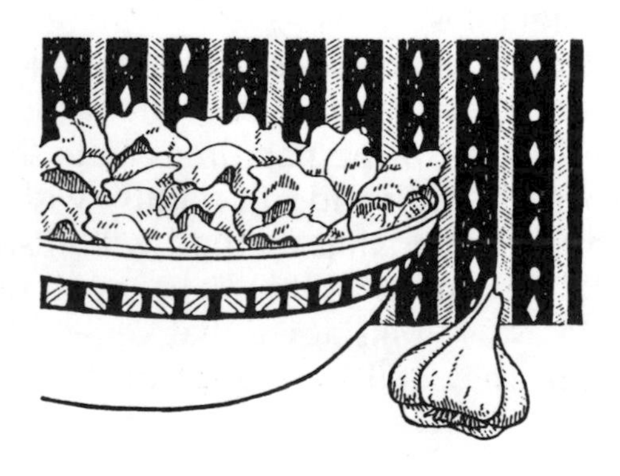

basic green salad

1/4 head lettuce, separated into leaves
juice of 2 lemons
1/4 cup sunflower or olive oil

Yield: 2 servings

1. Wash and dry the lettuce leaves.
2. Mix the lemon juice with the oil.
3. Drizzle over the lettuce leaves.
4. Toss.
5. Serve immediately.

variations

To liven up a green salad, you might add, to taste:
- Carrot and radish slices
- Cucumber slices and tomato slices
- Diced apple, parsley, and horseradish
- Finely chopped chicory
- Finely sliced red onion rings
- Grated beets and apple
- Grated carrot and paprika
- Raw endive, Swiss chard, or spinach

summer salad

1 large cucumber, peeled and cored
6 medium tomatoes
1 medium onion
1 medium green pepper, cored
1 medium red pepper, cored
2 cups cooked brown rice
juice of two lemons
4 tablespoons sunflower oil
4–5 large lettuce or spinach leaves

Yield: 5 cups

1. Chop the cucumber, tomatoes, onion, green pepper, and red pepper.
2. Combine in a large bowl.
3. In a separate bowl, mix the lemon juice and sunflower oil.
4. Pour the lemon/oil mixture over the vegetables.
5. Toss.
6. Add the cooked brown rice and toss again.
7. Refrigerate for 1 hour.
8. Turn the mixture out on a chilled serving dish lined with the lettuce or spinach leaves.
9. Serve cool.

Salad Dressings

All salads cry out for dressing. The basic lemon/oil dressing recipe that follows offers virtually unlimited opportunities to cooks with a bit of imagination. Following the lemon/oil recipe is a recipe for Moerman Mayonnaise. Made with egg yolks, this mayonnaise is a good basis for several tasty additions. These additions follow the basic mayonnaise recipe.

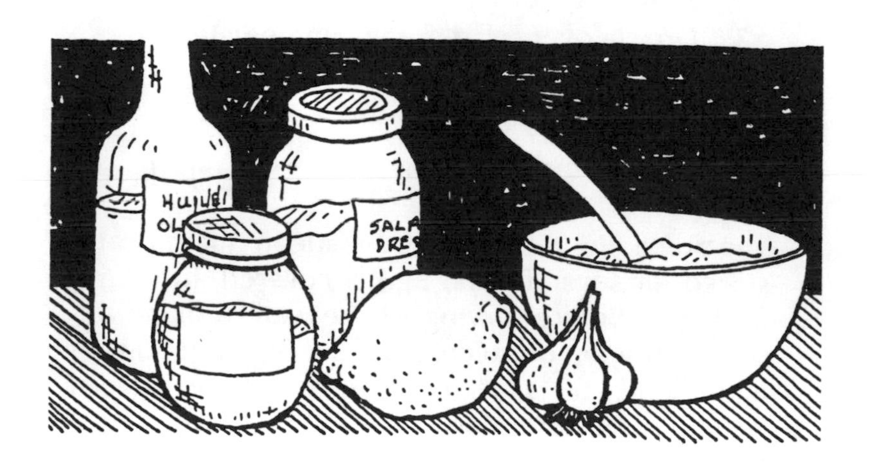

lemon/oil dressing

3 tablespoons sunflower or olive oil
1 tablespoon lemon juice

Yield: 1 serving

1. Combine oil and lemon juice in a small covered container.
2. Shake vigorously.
3. Drizzle over salad greens immediately after shaking.

variations

The preceding recipe can be made in quantity and stored for several days, tightly covered, in the refrigerator. Before serving, shake well to blend the oil and the lemon juice. Add any of the following ingredients, to taste, to create your own special version of this dressing.

- Chopped basil, chives, dill, oregano, parsley, rosemary, or thyme
- Chopped garlic or onion
- Crushed vegetable bouillon cube
- Grated cheese
- Honey

moerman mayonnaise

2 egg yolks
1 tablespoon lemon juice
1 teaspoon honey
1 cup sunflower oil

Yield: 1 1/2 cups

1. Have all ingredients at room temperature.
2. In a small mixing bowl, with an electric beater set on medium speed, beat the egg yolks, the lemon juice, and the honey.
3. Add 1/4 cup of the oil, one drop at a time, beating constantly.
4. Slowly add remaining oil, beating well until the mixture reaches a thick consistency.
5. Store, tightly covered, in the refrigerator for up to 1 week.

variations

To add variety to your mayonnaise, simply mix with one or more of the following, to taste:

- Chopped cucumber
- Chopped garlic

- Chopped green or red pepper
- Chopped onion
- Chopped parsley
- Chopped tomato
- Lemon juice
- Orange juice

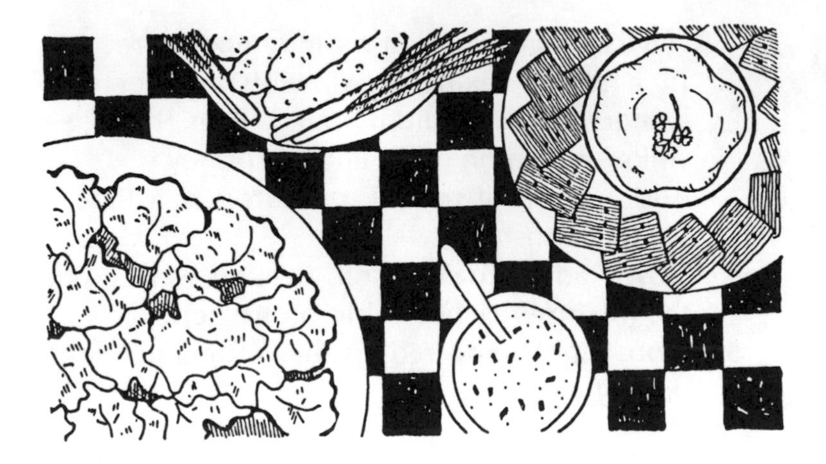

Sauces

Sauces, such as those that follow, are hearty complements to simple main dishes of cooked brown rice and vegetables. With a little imagination, you can create your own favorites.

onion sauce

2 cups vegetable broth
2 medium onions, finely chopped
1/2 cup corn flour mixed with 1/4 cup water
1/4 cup sunflower oil

Yield: 2 cups

1. Bring the broth to a boil, add the onions, and cook for 5 minutes.
2. Add the flour-and-water mixture to the broth.
3. Stir until well blended.
4. Remove from heat.
5. Add the oil after the sauce has cooled a bit.
6. Stir to blend.
7. Serve immediately.

cheese sauce

2 cups vegetable broth
1/2 cup corn flour
1/4 cup grated cheese
1/4 cup sunflower oil

Yield: 2 cups

1. Bring the broth to a boil; add the flour and stir until the mixture is well blended.
2. Remove from heat, add the grated cheese and the oil.
3. Stir well.
4. Serve immediately.

variations

The preceding recipe may be varied by substituting 1/4 cup of any chopped herb for the cheese. Add the herbs after the sauce has been removed from the heat. Let the sauce rest for 1–2 minutes so that the flavors can blend. Then, serve.

tomato sauce

2 cups water
4 large tomatoes, peeled and chopped
1 large onion, chopped
1 vegetable bouillon cube
1-2 tablespoons whole grain flour
1/4 cup olive oil

Yield: 2 cups

1. Bring the water, the tomatoes, the onion, and the vegetable bouillon to a boil in a covered stock pot.
2. Add the flour, stirring well, to thicken the sauce.
3. Remove from heat, add the olive oil, stir to blend.
4. Serve immediately.

variations

The preceding recipe may be varied by adding 1/4 cup of grated cheese to the sauce as it cooks or 2 egg yolks to the sauce after it has been removed from the heat. Blend well. Serve immediately.

milk sauce

2 cups low-fat milk
3 tablespoons whole grain flour
pinch sea salt
1 teaspoon nutmeg
1 tablespoon butter

Yield: 2 cups

1. Bring the low-fat milk and the salt to a boil in a covered stock pot.
2. Add the flour, stirring well, to thicken the sauce.
3. Add the nutmeg and the butter to the thickened sauce.
4. Stir well.
5. Serve immediately.

Main Dishes

The wealth of whole grains and whole grain pastas available at the supermarket today make it easy to experiment with satisfying main dish menus like the ones that follow. Serve these with freshly steamed vegetables, green salads, whole grain breads, and fruit desserts for nutritious, satisfying main-dish meals.

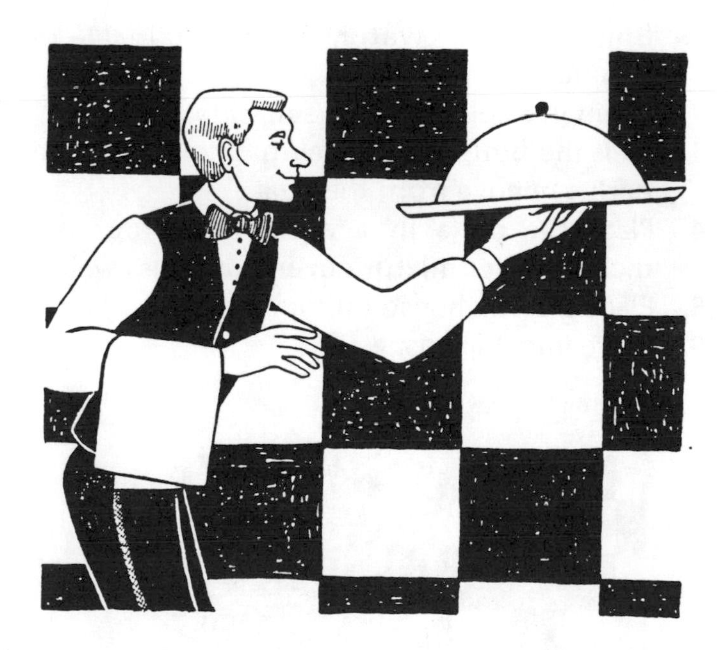

whole grain pasta with garden herbs

1 cup uncooked whole grain pasta
4 cups water
2 tablespoons butter
1/4 cup chopped parsley
1/4 cup chopped basil
1/3 cup grated cheese

Yield: 1 main-dish serving

1. Boil pasta in water, uncovered, 11–13 minutes.
2. Strain in a colander and set aside.
3. Melt the butter in a small pan; mix with the herbs; remove from the heat.
4. Place the pasta in a warm dish. Pour the melted butter mixture over it and toss well.
5. Place grated cheese on top.
6. Serve immediately.

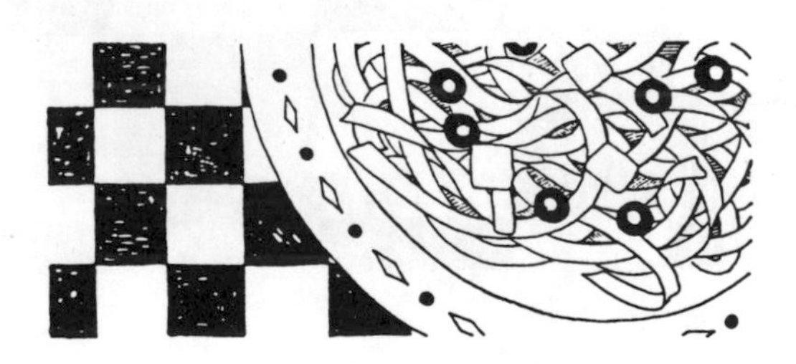

paella with mixed vegetables

1 cup uncooked brown rice
1 bay leaf
1 tablespoon butter
1 red pepper, cored and chopped
1 small onion, diced
1 clove garlic, chopped
2 cups raw, sliced vegetables of your choice (eggplant, zucchini, whole peas, spinach, and/or broccoli)
2 diced tomatoes
dash pepper

Yield: 2 main-dish servings

1. Cook the brown rice according to directions, adding the bay leaf to the cooking water.
2. When the rice is done, remove the bay leaf and discard; cover the rice, and set aside.
3. Melt the butter in a large pan and sauté the pepper, the onion, and the garlic in it.
4. Add the mixed vegetables, cover, and cook over low heat for 3–4 minutes.
5. Add the rice, the tomatoes, and the pepper.
6. Mix well.
7. Serve immediately.

whole wheat pizza

1/2 cup warm water
2 tablespoons olive oil
1 teaspoon honey
2 teaspoons dry yeast
1 1/4 cups whole wheat flour
3–4 large tomatoes, diced
1 small onion, diced
1 medium green or red pepper, cored and diced (optional)
1/2 cup grated cheese
1 teaspoon basil
1 teaspoon parsley
2 teaspoons oregano

Yield: 1, 12 1/2-inch, round pizza pie

1. Combine the water, the milk, the honey, and the yeast and let stand for about 10 minutes to allow the yeast to dissolve.
2. Add 1 cup of the flour and mix well.
3. Knead in the remaining flour. The dough will be soft and slightly sticky.
4. Place this dough in a lightly oiled bowl; turn over to oil on both sides; cover with a damp cloth and let rise until it doubles in bulk, about 1 hour.

5. Transfer the dough to an oiled cookie sheet or pizza pan.
6. Using your hands, flatten and stretch the dough to cover the pan in an even thickness.
7. Cover the dough with the tomatoes, the onion, the pepper, the cheese, the basil, the parsley, and the oregano.
8. Bake in a preheated 350°F oven for 20–30 minutes, or until the topping is hot and the crust is browned.
9. Slice and serve immediately.

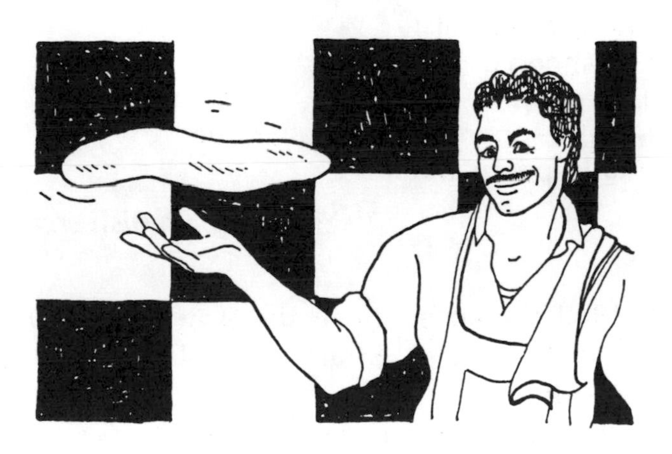

whole grain spaghetti with fresh vegetable sauce

4 oz. whole grain spaghetti, uncooked
(approximately 1/4 of a 1-lb. box)
4 cups water
1 large tomato, chopped
2 medium onions, chopped
1 clove garlic, minced
1 tablespoon chopped parsley
1 teaspoon basil
1 teaspoon oregano
dash pepper
1-2 tablespoons whole grain flour
4 tablespoons water

Yield: 1 main-dish serving

1. Boil the spaghetti in the water, uncovered, 11–13 minutes. Strain in a colander and set aside.
2. Melt the butter in a small pan.
3. Saute the tomato, the onions, the garlic, the parsley, the basil, the oregano, and the pepper, covered, for 5 minutes.
4. Add the flour to the water and blend until no lumps remain.

5. Add this mixture to the vegetable mixture and blend well to thicken.
6. Continue cooking for 1 minute.
7. Place the spaghetti on a warm dish, pour the sauce over the spaghetti, and serve immediately.

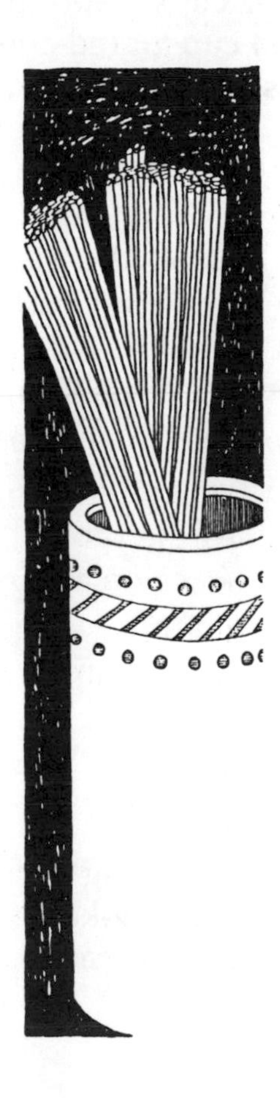

brown rice and vegetables

1/2 cup uncooked brown rice
1 tablespoon butter
1/4 cup water
1–2 cups assorted diced vegetables
1/4 cup grated cheese
assorted chopped herbs, to taste

Yield: 1 main-dish serving

1. Cook the rice according to package directions; set aside.
2. Cook the vegetables, covered, in the water for 2–3 minutes.
3. Add the butter, the herbs, and the rice to the vegetables.
4. Mix gently.
5. Place on a warm dish and sprinkle the cheese on top.
6. Serve immediately.

variations

The preceding recipe can be varied, substituting for the uncooked brown rice any uncooked whole grains: oats, barley, rye, wheat, or buckwheat.

whole grain noodle-spinach casserole

1 cup uncooked whole grain noodles
4 cups water
1 cup fresh spinach, chopped
1/3 cup water
1 tablespoon butter at room temperature
1 tablespoon whole grain flour
1/4 cup low-fat milk
1/4 cup grated cheese
dash nutmeg
dash pepper

Yield: 1 main-dish serving

1. Boil the noodles in water, uncovered, 11–13 minutes.
2. Strain in a colander and place in an ovenproof casserole.
3. Cook the spinach briefly, until wilted, in the 1/3 cup water, strain, and place in a layer on top of the noodles.
4. Mix the butter, the flour, the milk, and the cheese.
5. Pour over the spinach.
6. Sprinkle the nutmeg and pepper over the top.

7. Bake, uncovered, in a preheated 350°F oven for 10 minutes.
8. Serve immediately.

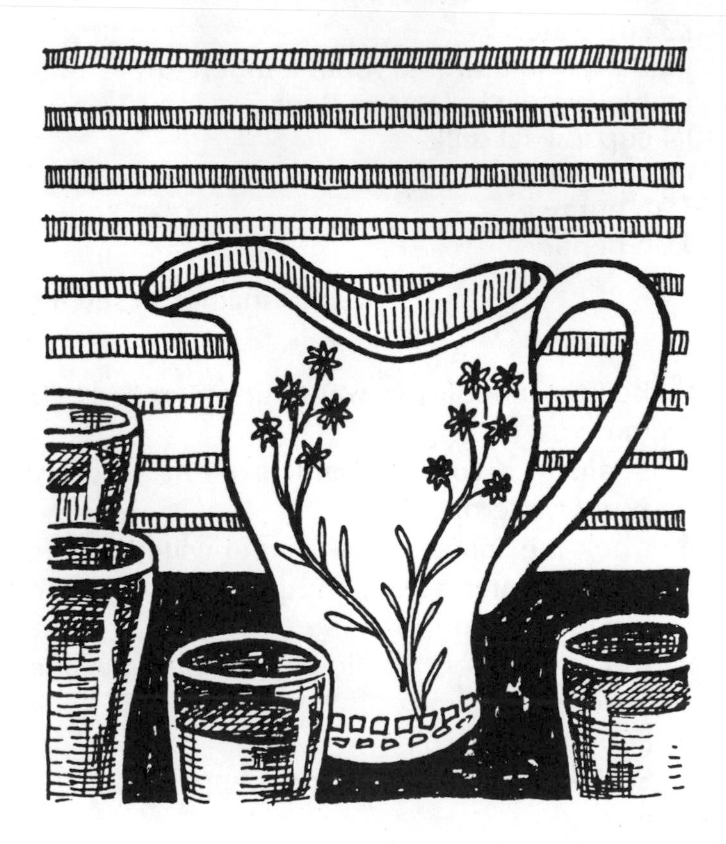

Beverages

Buttermilk, low-fat, and herb teas may all be enjoyed on the Moerman Diet. However, the most important beverages on the diet are made from the fresh juices of vegetables and fruits. The ideal fruits and vegetables to juice are those that are fresh, organically grown, and in season. Do not juice canned or frozen fruits or vegetables. To prepare fruits and vegetables for juicing, wash and trim them well.

Using a hand juicer, an inexpensive electric juice-extracting machine, and/or a blender, you can concoct your own favorite juice beverages. Enjoy these throughout the day: alone; mixed with spring water, buttermilk, or other juices; or blended with whole fruits. All of the suggested beverage ingredients that follow are to be blended in equal proportions. Each combination yields one serving; feel free to double or triple the ingredients to make more servings, as long as they are consumed immediately. You may vary the ingredients and proportions as you wish, according to the guidelines of the Moerman Diet.

drink combinations

These healthful combinations are energy boosters. Serve cold for best flavor.

- Buttermilk and apple, lemon, orange, or strawberry juice

- Buttermilk and egg yolk
- Buttermilk, beet juice, and lemon juice
- Buttermilk, pineapple juice, and apple or lemon juice

juice combinations

These wholesome combinations offer variety. Some are sweet; some are tangy. They all taste great.

- Alfalfa sprout, beet, radish
- Carrot, apple and/or pineapple
- Grape, apple, lemon
- Green pepper, cucumber, lettuce, red pepper
- Prune, apple, pear
- Spinach, carrot, parsley, tomato
- Tomato, cabbage, carrot, cucumber, red pepper, scallion, spinach
- Tomato, carrot, onion
- Watermelon, including seeds and rind

blender shakes

Try freezing the fruits below before blending them together to make frosty treats.

- Banana, strawberry, orange
- Cherry, peach, pear
- Grapefruit, grape, orange, honey, and two egg yolks
- Grapefruit, orange, and two egg yolks
- Honeydew, cantaloupe, strawberry
- Pineapple, apple, and buttermilk

Desserts

Desserts need not be dull just because a nutritional program is therapeutic. In fact, a tasty diet that also makes you well allows you to get more from life. That's what the Moerman Therapy is all about: feeling better so that you can enjoy life. Dr. Moerman believed that dessert time should be a time of enjoyment. In keeping with his wishes, the recipes that follow are fun to prepare and to eat. Feel free to vary the ingredients and proportions of the foods allowed on the diet according to your own tastes and preferences to create your own special desserts.

rödgröt
strawberry delight

2 cups crushed strawberries
4 cups water
1/4 cup uncooked, ground brown rice
2 tablespoons honey
1/2 cup yogurt

Yield: 4–6 servings

1. Bring the water to a boil in an uncovered stock pot.
2. Add the ground brown rice, the crushed strawberries, and the honey.
3. Allow this mixture to boil thoroughly, stirring constantly, until it forms a custard-like consistency, approximately 8–10 minutes.
4. Cool and refrigerate.
5. Serve cold in small dishes. Garnish each serving with a dollop of yogurt.

variations

To vary the preceding recipe, you may use the crushed berries and unsweetened applesauce in the following proportions instead of the crushed strawberries called for in the preceding recipe.

- 1 cup blackberries and 1 cup unsweetened applesauce
- 1 cup blueberries and 1 cup unsweetened applesauce
- 1 cup strawberries and 1 cup black currants
- 1 cup strawberries and 1 cup unsweetened applesauce
- 2 cups blackberries
- 2 cups blueberries

hearty cheese cake

2 1/2 cups corn flour
1 cup butter
1/2 cup grated cheese
2 egg yolks
1 teaspoon celery salt

Yield: 1 cake

1. Melt the butter in an uncovered stock pot.
2. Slowly add the grated cheese, the corn flour, the celery salt, and the egg yolks.
3. Mix well.
4. Remove from heat.
5. Allow to rest, covered, for 1 hour.
6. Roll the dough out to a 1/2-inch thickness.
7. Then roll, jelly-roll fashion, into a long tube shape.
8. Press the two ends of the tube together to form a circular shape.
9. Place on a lightly oiled cookie sheet.
10. Bake in a preheated 350°F oven for 15 minutes.
11. Serve warm or at room temperature.

basic recipe fruit cocktail

2 cups diced fruit
1 cup fruit juice

Yield: 2–4 servings

1. Chill all ingredients.
2. Combine diced fruit and fruit juice.
3. Serve in stem glasses.

variations

The preceding recipe can be varied according to whatever fruits are in season. Some suggestions follow:

- diced melon, diced apples, and diced pears mixed with grape juice
- diced pineapple, diced apples, and sliced bananas mixed with grape juice
- whole strawberries and whole, pitted cherries mixed with diced apples and apple juice

fruit bread

5 cups whole wheat flour
1 teaspoon sea salt
1/4 cup honey
1/2 cup grated carrots
1/2 cup chopped apples
1/2 cup raisins
1 tablespoon cinnamon
1 teaspoon nutmeg
1 cup lukewarm, low-fat milk
3 teaspoons dried yeast or 6 teaspoons fresh yeast

Yield: 1 loaf

1. Mix the flour with the salt.
2. Mix the honey, the carrots, the apples, the raisins, the cinnamon, and the nutmeg with the low-fat milk.
3. Dissolve the yeast in half the milk mixture and wait until it has a good, frothy head on it.
4. Add this mixture to the remaining milk mixture and add to the flour mixture.
5. Mix thoroughly to form a soft dough.
6. Knead for 5 minutes.
7. Put the dough in a warm place and leave it until it has doubled in size, about 1–2 hours.
8. Knead a second time.

9. Place in a lightly buttered bread pan. Leave to rise in the pan for approximately 1/2 hour.
10. Bake at 400°F 40 minutes, until the loaf sounds hollow when knocked on the bottom.
11. Do not over-bake.
12. Cool, slice, and serve with cream cheese.

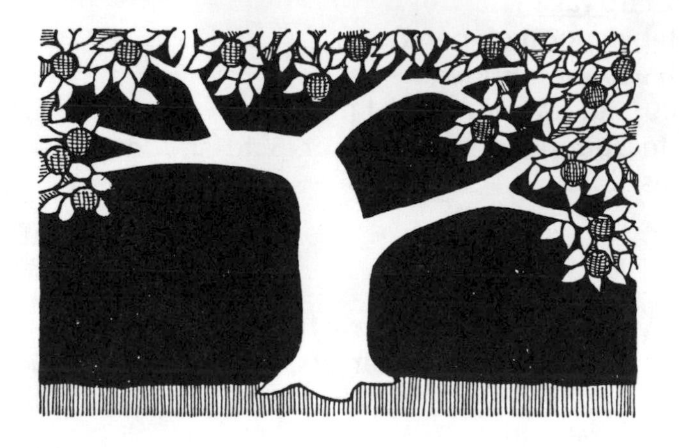

baked pears

2 large, firm pears
1/4 cup water
1 teaspoon cinnamon

Yield: 2–4 servings

1. Peel, core, and halve the pears.
2. Pour the water in the bottom of a shallow baking dish.
3. Place pears, flat side down, in the baking dish.
4. Sprinkle cinnamon over pears.
5. Bake, uncovered, in a preheated 350°F oven for 8–10 minutes.
6. Serve warm.

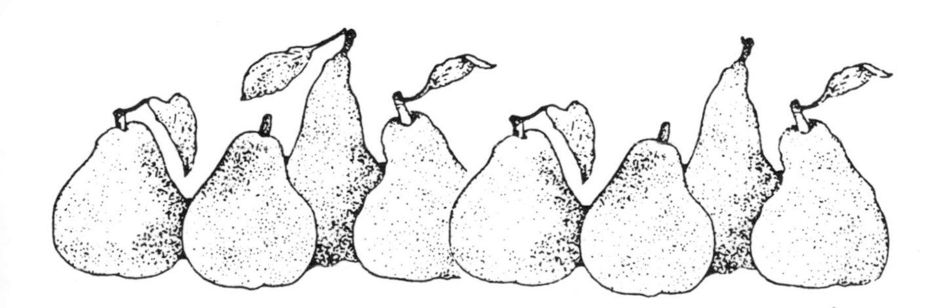

A Recipe for Good Health

Having read—and cooked—your way through the preceding recipes, you can now see that the Moerman Diet is economical, flexible, and good tasting. However, it is important to remember that the most significant recipe in the Moerman Therapy is the one for beating cancer. It includes equal parts of determination, to stick to the diet and supplementation program; positive thinking, to overcome any doubts that might be present; and love and support, from those with whom you work and live. As the case histories of hundreds of cured cancer patients attest, this recipe works. Now, it's up to you to use it for your own successful recovery. Good luck! And good health!

Glossary

antibody	A blood protein with the power to combine specifically with a molecule or group of atoms.
antigen	A molecule that has the power to produce antibody molecules.
benign tumor	A tumor that is non-invasive and non-malignant.
biopsy	The excision of tissue for microscopic examination to establish diagnosis.
cancer	Any of the various types of malignant neoplasms characterized by an uncontrolled proliferation of cells.
carcinogen	Any cancer-producing substance or condition.

carcinoma A malignant tumor of epithelial or endothelial origin.

chemotherapy A cancer treatment that uses a specific chemical agent to arrest the progress of, or eradicate, cancer without causing irreversible injury to healthy tissues. Chemotherapeutic agents are administered mainly by oral, intramuscular and intravenous routes, and are distributed through the bloodstream. Their side effects include nausea, vomiting, hair loss, pain, and weight loss.

chromosome A collection of genes and supporting structures in the nucleus of a cell.

colon The large bowel extending from the cecum to the rectum. In its various parts it has appropriate names: ascending colon, descending colon, transverse colon, sigmoid colon. A diet high in meat, salt, processed foods, sugar, and white flour can, over a period of time, lead to cancer of the colon.

DNA Deoxyribonucleic acid, the self-replicating substance of genes.

encapsulation The walling-off or enclosing of fibrous tissues.

endoscope The general term for those diagnostic procedures that use a tube-shaped, long, metal scope to view any of the various body cavities and or organs. Permits examination, photography, and biopsy of most of the organs of the body.

enzyme A protein secreted by cells that acts as a catalyst to increase (or decrease) the rate of a chemical reaction, without itself being changed.

epithelium An outer layer of cells covering the skin and other surfaces.

gene The functioning unit of

heredity, consisting of a chain of nucleotides (the units of DNA).

hemoglobin The iron-containing, red-pigmented part of red blood cells. It combines with, and produces, oxygen in the blood, which is then transported throughout the body via the bloodstream.

hormone A glandular secretion carried by the bloodstream to the organs that it regulates.

hormone therapy A form of cancer treatment that either regulates or administers hormones. Used primarily to treat cancers of the lymphatic system, breast, and prostate.

immunotherapy A form of cancer treatment that seeks to eradicate the disease by strengthening the body's own immune system.

interferon A natural protein used in immunotherapy, effective against virtually every known virus. When the DNA core of a virus invades a cell, it triggers the cell's defense production of interferon. Cancer researchers are working on developing an artificial interferon inducer to make interferon before an attack of cancer to protect the cell.

laparascopy — A diagnostic procedure using a long, thin metal scope that is inserted through a small abdominal incision to view the pelvic organs. Used for biopsy, aspiration of cysts, photography, and division of adhesions.

leucocyte — Any one of the white blood cells (granulocytes or lymphocytes).

leukemia — A cancerous blood disease in which white cells are abnormal in type or number. Classification is according to the type of leucocyte found and whether the condition is acute or chronic. This form of cancer is systemic, rather than arising from tissues like solid tumor cancers.

lymphocyte A lymph cell (white blood cell) formed in the lymphatic system and eventually emptied into the venous circulation.

macrophage A larger cell with the ability to destroy bacteria.

malignant tumor A tumor that has invaded surrounding tissue.

mammography The X-ray examination of one or both breasts after injection of opaque dye. Used to determine if cancer is present.

melanoma A tumor that forms from the pigment- producing cells of the deeper layers in the skin, or of the eye.

metabolism The sum of the chemical reactions involved in the function of nutrition.

metastasis A term describing the action of secondary tumors that appear in parts of the body remote from the site of the primary tumor as a result of bloodborne or lymphatic spread.

myeloma — A primary malignant tumor of bone marrow; most frequently multiple.

necrosis — The death of cells, tissues, or organs.

neoplasm — A new growth or tumor, either benign or malignant.

neuroblastoma — A malignant brain tumor arising in the adrenal medulla from tissue of the sympathetic nervous system.

nitrosamines — Cancer-causing compounds found in pickled foods, cured meats, and in the stomach when nitrites react with amino acids from the proteins in foods. Vitamin C destroys nitrosamines.

oncology — The scientific study of tumors.

osteoporosis — A condition that causes reduction in the mineral content of bone.

rectoscope	A long, tubular metal instrument used to examine the rectum.
remission	A period of abatement of a disease.
sarcoma	A malignant tumor of connective tissue, bone, or muscle.
surgery	A form of cancer treatment in which the cancerous tumor is removed.
terminal	A term used by mainstream physicians to classify cancer cases that are viewed as untreatable through mainstream methods.
tissue	A collection of similar cells and the intercellular substance surrounding them.
T-lymphocyte	A lymphocyte produced (programmed) by the thymus.
toximolecular	A term used to describe the action of molecules that exert a toxic or poi-

sonous action, as with most drugs.

tumor A mass of abnormal tissue that resembles the normal tissues in structure but fulfils no useful function and grows at the expense of the body.

X-ray therapy A form of cancer treatment using short rays of the electromagnetic spectrum in high doses to destroy cancerous tissue.

Index

N

O

P

R

S

T

V

W